COLLEGE BASIC TRAINING

Strengthen your mind and body to leap any college hurdle

SUSAN JENSEN

ISBNs: 978-0-9905789-2-5 (print)
         978-0-9905789-3-2 (ebook)

Editor: Mary Stewart Swanson, Ph.D.

Cover design and photo: Jill Gardiner

Book design: Patti Frazee

Exercise photos: Dani Werner

Images: used by permission from Shutterstock, Inc.

~Swan Fitness Publishing~

To my children,
Shaylee and Tanner Jensen

Acknowledgments

I want to thank all of the young adults, including my children, who have reached out to me, shared personal stories, and made me aware of the concerns that many young people deal with upon entering college. A special thanks to Shaylee and Tanner Jensen for taking the time to read my manuscript, giving me honest opinions, and showing an inexhaustible enthusiasm for this project.

Mary Stewart Swanson, my mom, has contributed unwavering support and meticulous editing. I could not have completed this book without her. Sincere thanks, also, to Jill Gardiner, a dear friend and sister-in-law extraordinaire, for believing in my written word, being my cheerleader, and enthusiastically joining my creative team.

Patti Frazee, my book designer, deserves special thanks for listening intently to my ideas, experimenting with new technology, and turning my personal vision into an even better reality.

Finally, I want to extend heartfelt thanks to Corey Jensen, my husband and the love of my life, for his constant patience, love and support, even when he had to compete with my computer for a date!

Table of Contents

COLLEGE
BASIC TRAINING

INTRODUCTION

Maybe you are a senior in high school and noticing some changes in your body: jeans are tight, the tummy is a little thicker, and you think to yourself, "What is happening to me? This is not OK!" Or perhaps you are a freshman in college who walked in with what others may have described as a "rockin' body," and by the time the holidays roll around you look at pictures and see that your face resembles a balloon, and your thighs are rubbing together more than ever.

On the other hand, you might be someone who has never had a weight issue in your life and vows that the "freshman fifteen" is not going to happen to you! Yet you feel a little anxiety about all the responsibilities and temptations that go along with college life.

Regardless of your situation, the goal is not perfection in behavior or appearance. The goal is to maintain a healthy lifestyle that leads to a healthy mind, healthy body and healthy body image.

Let's get straight to the point. College is a big change. As a freshman you might find yourself in a tiny dorm room with enough space to turn your body around 360 degrees and, if you are lucky, perform a leg lift—as long as you are the only one in the room! The fridge, if you even have one, is big enough to hold a couple of bottles of water and a piece of deli meat. Then you venture out to the campus cafeteria, which does offer a salad bar, but of course it's next to the chicken tenders, greasy hamburgers, French fries and ice cream machine! Can you say "willpower" or "temptation"?

Soon you discover partying with your friends, which includes late nights, high-calorie beverages and the two a.m. feedings consisting of munchies like pizza and chicken wings. You wake up the next morning sleep deprived, and it's all you can do to muster up the energy to go to class or hit the books. The gym rarely fits into this equation! A few weeks in, and the first freshman virus hits: you're down and out with a fever, sore throat and body aches. You're behind in school, and it's all you can do to get through this week of illness hell!

Eventually, a light bulb goes on and you discover your diet is full of fat and unhealthy carbs. Maybe you have even turned to some kind of stimulant to get by. Your exercise habits are almost nonexistent, and a full night's sleep is nearly impossible. Stress sets in as you approach midterms, and you realize you completely suck at time management! Not to mention you are still trying to figure out how to do laundry, keep your room picked up so your roommate doesn't murder you, figure out who your group of friends are, and find a way to manage your money since you realize you have only five dollars left to get you through the rest of the week. This is called transition and can be a complete shock to your mind and body!

Let's not forget that as a college student, you have much to celebrate and look forward to. This is your time in life to find unique paths, make your own decisions, build your dreams, and have a blast doing it! We all know that pursuing higher education is one of the most positive avenues we can take: our intellectual training prepares us to achieve great things, and the life experiences of college provide steppingstones to individuality, lifelong relationships and independence.

However, outside pressures, impulses, temptations or naivety can throw a wrench into our plans and derail us from our road to success. We can't control everything, but the more knowledge and awareness we have about our physical, mental and emotional well-being, the better off we will be when making our own decisions and helping others with similar issues.

I want to bring positive awareness, promote healthy minds and bodies, enhance life, be a resource for help, and perhaps even prevent a tragedy.

Throughout my career as a Personal Fitness Trainer and Health Coach, I have found great satisfaction in helping people of all ages with diet, exercise, motivation, self-control and life balance. More importantly, I am the mom of two young adults who are college students. Throughout the brief lives of both my daughter and son I have seen their joys, their struggles, their excitement and their pain.

I have the same passion for helping my clients as I do for helping my kids and their friends. I want to share my life experiences and professional knowledge with you to help make your life transition into college a positive one. Let me empower you with strength and knowledge, engage you with some humor, encourage you to achieve moderation and balance, and motivate you with inspirational stories.

CHAPTER 1
Media Distraction and Time Management

How you manage your minutes and hours will make or break you—no joke.

When my neighbor's son first moved into a college dorm a hundred miles from home, he could hardly contain himself. Freedom, independence, parties, cute girls, new friends, no parental nagging!

He forgot about all the times his mom had bailed him out when he was living at home. When he lost his keys, she had helped him get new ones, awakened him when his alarm didn't go off, and edited his papers and fixed his printer minutes before his assignments were due.

He was surprised to see that clean, folded clothes don't magically appear weekly and that access to food could often be a problem in his dorm. He had to be bummed when he realized he couldn't skip a test he wasn't ready for because his mom wasn't there to bail him out with a note. When he became sleep deprived and sick from pulling all-nighters, he had no one to supply him with medicine or make his doctor appointments, either. Also, he learned that leaving his clothes all over the floor didn't fly in a 10'x10' dorm room he shared with someone else. Moms will usually forgive you, but a roommate may kill you or, at the very least, abandon you next semester!

Highs and lows during college are abundant for most students. Juggling challenging class work, friends, and work or group involvement can be overwhelming. If you couple that with sleep deprivation, drug or alcohol use, and poor eating habits, life can reach an all-time low.

Those who like structure and organization probably fare pretty well, but for many young people, being organized, managing time, and handling media distraction is a big challenge. Some of the tricks to managing stress might seem obvious, but until you actually try them, you won't be convinced they can change your entire college experience for the better. In addition, your GPA will be lookin' good!

My goal is for you to be healthy, happy and successful! Disorganization can lead to a really unhealthy life that may include sleep deprivation, anxiety, depression and low self-esteem. People who don't develop decent study and time management skills usually struggle to fit in the components of life that add to our wellness, such as attention to healthy eating and exercise.

Although this topic is not very exciting and engaging, learning how to make an efficient plan is one of the first things you must do to be successful. If you're tempted to skip this chapter, do it at your own risk because it contains information that could make or break you in college and beyond!

Media distraction or obsession

Girls, are you constantly looking for that next photo you can post on Instagram with your cute friends? Is that tray of sushi too irresistibly beautiful not to show your Facebook community immediately? What about that steaming, creamy Caribou latte? Who wouldn't "like" that?

Does your boyfriend thrive on this unspoken competition between the bros on who can post the "sickest" photos or the funniest tweets? Oh, yeah, we all know the dudes love to get a reaction. Just remember, real men don't have to post photos of liquor bottles! You tell 'm girl!

Once the photo is up, are you obsessed with seeing how many "likes" you have? After it's been up for a while, are you anxious about whether your roots look bad or your forehead is too big? When you are at a family dinner or a meeting where you know it's not kosher to have your phone out, does feeling the "buzz" in your pocket make you anxious? Does it take all the willpower you have not to look at the phone screen? Or, when you don't have your phone on you, do you feel a phantom buzz?

How often do you totally miss parts of conversation or even noteworthy material from a school lecture because you're texting a friend about Thursday night's plans or checking Facebook? You may even be guilty of shopping on eBay during class. Now that's a distraction!

Have you ever bumped into someone while you were walking and texting? Or worse yet, walked into a moving vehicle? I'm sure this has happened somewhere. Do you hang out with your phone all night? Do you check it when you wake up at 4 a.m.? Or do you wake up at 4 a.m. because someone else is calling you with unnecessary drama they may or may not remember the next morning? Are your negative tweets not really messages to the world, but underlying communication to an X?

This is exhausting! I know not all students are deep into social media. However, if you are over-the-top interactive, such a preoccupation can have some serious, negative consequences. You may not even realize where you stand on the media-obsessed continuum. I strongly suggest you look at your habits closely and ask yourself these questions.

- How much time in a day do I spend messing with unproductive social media?
- Does it cause me anxiety?
- Do I miss segments of conversation because my phone distracts me?
- Is it causing me to be rude to my friends and family?
- When I'm trying to study or focus, is it getting in the way of my concentration?
- Is it feeding my procrastination?
- Am I using it for the wrong reasons?

SELFIE :)

- Is it affecting my sleep?
- When I am driving, am I compelled to look at my phone or constantly change the song from my play list?

Social media can be very stimulating, exciting and irresistible! Media addiction is not too dissimilar from drug and alcohol addiction. Some of us have a difficult time resisting things that make us feel good, no matter what the long-term consequences. For example, some people are able to have a couple of drinks or refrain from alcohol completely when it's necessary, but others feel the need to continuously sip on something regardless of their responsibilities. Can you put your phone away for extended periods of time when you study, or are you compelled to have it on, and near you at all hours of the day and night?

Anthony Wagner, co-author of a study done at Stanford University, states, "Each time we get a message or text, our dopamine reward circuits probably get activated, since the desire for social connection is so wired into us."[1] Dopamine is the "feel good" chemical, so it's no wonder some of us can't get off Instagram!

I know you think you are a great multi-tasker, but I'm not sure there is such a thing as even a good multi-tasker! The truth is no matter how good you think you are at doing two things with the same part of your brain at the same time, some information will go missing! Scientific evidence shows that students who are interrupted by media technology while studying aren't taking in the class material nearly as effectively as they could. The constant interruption causes the information received to become spotty or fragmented and not stored in the memory as deeply. Material recall is worse, and it is difficult to transfer the information to other contexts. Mistakes increase because the brain has to regroup and pick up where it left off before the interruption.[2]

I'll never forget the compassion I felt when a student told me a story about missing a very important presentation due to a brief distraction:

> *After learning a life lesson about bad attendance last semester, I was finally diligent about attending my entrepreneur class all this semester. In this class our grade was to be based on one project, which we worked on for two months. It included a final oral presentation.*
>
> *We concocted a business idea, and I helped pound out a detailed business plan. I personally put in long hours creating our website and Twitter account. We then carried out the duties of our creative service, which we were proud to share.*
>
> *Our big day finally came; I had stayed up all night to finish the last details*

of this important presentation and was exhausted. Business leaders from all over the community were coming to hear our ideas and determine if we might be worthy employees for their internship programs or businesses.

I was going to nail this! I struggled to find the most appropriate business attire and even put the iron to the shirt on my own! I was ready, so I thought. I walked into the lecture hall and saw my group finishing up our presentation.

It turns out that I missed a minor detail in class: we were scheduled to present one hour before the class period usually started! I turned white as a ghost and felt faint. WTF! My heart sank. I had let my whole team down and embarrassed myself in front of the most influential business leaders in the city. My instructor just shook his head at me, making the situation more horrifying!

Needless to say, my grade sucked in a class that I had put the most time into. I tend to learn a lot of things the hard way. I now realize that when I am in class I need to be "present" both mentally and physically. This mistake will haunt me for the rest of my life!

—Taylor, age 20

Dr. Larry Rosen, author and researcher of media distraction in our culture, has written a book called *iDisorder*. He defines iDisorder as "changes to your brain's ability to process information and your ability to relate to the world due to your daily use of media and technology resulting in signs and symptoms of psychological disorders—such as stress, sleeplessness, and a compulsive need to check in with all of your technology."[3]

Dr. Rosen describes studies that display how quickly students begin losing focus in the classroom. Other window screens open on nearby computers often distract students. Many answer texts and check social media sites throughout the class period: "We found that students who glanced at their Facebook page just once during a 15-minute study period performed worse than those who never looked at that page, and students who had more windows open on their computer lost more focus on their studying."[4]

This observation may not be earth-shattering news to you, but my point here is I want you to become aware of how much you might compromise your learning with media distraction. Socializing is important. However, a more productive way to include your fun with social media is to reward yourself a certain amount of time for this after you have studied or read for a specific number of minutes.

For example, you might tell yourself, "I'm going to read and take notes on Chapter One and then take a 10-minute break to check my emails and texts." Or you may tell yourself, "I am going to turn my phone off for two hours and knock off all of my homework before I check anything else on my phone or computer that is not related to my assignment."

Experiment with boundaries you set for yourself. If you are going to study, you might as well get more bang for your buck—not only by doing the work, but also by retaining the information with as much focus and brainpower as possible! Besides, you will get it done in half the time! Save the multi-tasking for later. Looking at YouTube videos and texting at the same time won't hurt you in the long run, but texting and trying to listen to a class lecture at the same time will!

Have you experienced "phantom vibrations syndrome," the feeling that your cell phone is vibrating when it really isn't? Some researchers have indicated that this phenomenon could be the result of anxiety experienced by those who aren't able to check their phones regularly.[5]

Some studies indicate that heavy cell phone and computer use is linked to increased stress, trouble sleeping and depression, as well. However, the most tragic epidemic going on is driving distraction. I'm not going to rattle off the escalating statistics of deaths due to texting and driving, but let me paint a clearer picture of what the consequences might be.

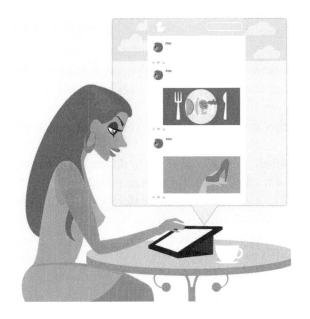

One second of distraction can kill you and an entire family. It's important that you take a moment to imagine yourself in a car accident. Feel the pain of a shattered leg and the horror of blood splattered everywhere, as your best friend lies limp and unconscious next to you. Envision yourself in therapy because you have had a severe brain injury and must learn to walk and talk again. Imagine how your parents would cope if they lost you. Picture family members of the children you killed because you felt compelled to respond to your boyfriend's text message.

Don't be selfish. Whenever you are tempted to text or search for the perfect song on your phone, think again! In fact, put your phone in the back seat. Finish up your communication before you start the engine. If you need to make a call, pull over to a safe parking lot. Pick your music before you back up out of the driveway, and settle for whatever song comes on next! Keep both hands on the wheel and both eyes on the road. No song or text is worth an injury or a life!

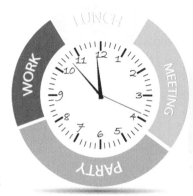

Time Management

Have a plan

Having a plan for managing your time at the very beginning of your freshman year is imperative for success and stress reduction. When you land in the dorms your freshman year, your time seems unlimited because you are in class only a few hours a day. After all, you had a seven-hour class schedule in high school. However, in college, unless you are involved in sports or other structured activities, you have much time to manage effectively and independently.

No mom or dad will be reminding you where you need to be and when. No adult will be eyeballing you until you pull the books out or calling you to get home when a paper is due or an exam scheduled. This huge responsibility lands on a young person all at once.

I've heard too many stories of freshmen who got lost in the parties at college, forgot the academics, and had to move home to pull themselves together. You may be stoked for that party, but if you don't have a good plan to balance the fun and the academics, the wind could be taken out of your sails!

Effective time management will decrease stress and anxiety, enabling you to get the best grades possible. If you truly want to grasp the material fully, plan to study two to three hours for every hour you spend in class. That calls for a lot of time management. Carrying a full class load in college can require as much time as having a full-time job!

Semester calendar

Gather all the syllabuses and other information you get the first week of class and visually organize your entire semester on a calendar. Map out your class schedule by recording class times, dates of quizzes and exams, dates that papers are due, meetings and other commitments to sports, work or other activities.

This process will give you an overview of the entire timeline. A view of this semester calendar will allow you visually comprehend all the weeks to come and make those days of "crunch time" very visible so that you can better prepare in the weeks preceding them.

Monthly calendar

A monthly calendar allows you to plot out and organize your weeks, so that you can plan for the amount of time you will need for reading, note taking, studying, writing and editing. Don't hesitate to ask your instructor to suggest time allotments so that you can better prepare.

Weekly calendar

Taking 20 minutes to create a weekly calendar will save you much time in the long run. This weekly plan will cut out the extra time you spend trying to decide which task to accomplish first. If you have a Mac or Google calendar, which is free, you can print out a weekly calendar using i-cal. A weekly planner will allow you to plan all the details you need to do. Put this visual reminder in a place that will enable you see it regularly—your fridge or in your notebook.

If you record lab times, meal times, study times and all personal activities and commitments, you will stay on task. Think about what times of day your brain works best for studying. Then prioritize the tasks you need to accomplish.[6]

Helpful hints

- **Make use of short, unscheduled time slots.** It's amazing how using short increments of time can add up to a lot of completed tasks. Use that extra 15 minutes any time you get it, even between classes!

- **Refer to a piece of paper or email once.** Instead of shuffling piles of paper back and forth, decide what to do with each page and be done! That goes for emails, too: read and respond immediately.

- **Schedule some personal time.** Relationships, exercise, sleep and a little bit of fun are important, so make sure to build them into your schedule. If you are ahead of the time-line, reward yourself.

- **Deal with your distraction.** If something is bothering you, it's best to deal with it and move on so that it doesn't throw you completely off track.

- **Try to be consistent about your study times and locations.** A little structure will save you a lot of time in the long run. If you know where you are going to study and have regular time slots, you will prevent a lot of wasted time trying to figure it out.

- **Review ASAP.** If you review material shortly after it has been presented to you, you will enhance your retention and accuracy.

- **Limit study time.** Concentrate for one and a half to two hours at a time when your concentration is best. After that, returns are diminished. Take a break and switch gears to another course.

- **Prioritize what needs to be done first.** If some of those most urgent tasks are your least favorite, that's good because getting the toughest things out of the way is a great stress reliever!

- **Double your time.** Believe it or not, most estimated time allotments for homework fall short! Doubling the time you think you will need to complete a task is much more realistic.[7]

- **When setting up your schedule, stick by even your toughest decisions.** There are always times when it is best to pass on that social invitation. Go with your gut, have the willpower to do what you need to do, and reap the rewards!

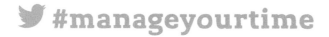 **#manageyourtime**

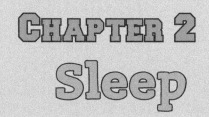

CHAPTER 2
Sleep

**Get on the road to weight and
health maintenance, good grades,
and improved social life.**

We need sleep for many reasons, both mentally and physically. In addition to causing severe stress and other ailments, sleep deprivation doubles the risk of obesity! We might think that the less we sleep, the more calories we will burn and the more weight we will lose, but research shows quite the opposite. As a result of hormonal, appetite-stimulating changes, sleep deprivation can lead to weight gain.[8] Who wants that?

Are you a person who stays up until three in the morning watching YouTube videos or getting hung up on Twitter? Or maybe you do your homework with the relaxed attitude that it's no big deal to stay up all night because you have two hours between classes to catch up on your shut-eye? Or do you sleep with your phone on your chest in case you get that emergency call in the middle of the night or (let's be realistic) that drunk dial or text that is so incredibly important?

Ask yourself this: how important is it to get a text from someone who won't even remember they texted you? Ummm, let's take that phone-on-the-chest off the priority list. Shut off your phone, and charge it away from your bed!

How realistic is it for a college student to get eight to ten hours of solid sleep a night? In your dreams: no pun intended. But the reality is that you will not be well rested if you break up your sleep segments. Research shows that getting longer periods of uninterrupted sleep is far more beneficial than getting a few hours of sleep and then taking naps. So do what you can to get that full night's sleep. Your physical body and the emotions and focus coming from your brain will function at a much higher level. In addition, you might fend off those nasty viruses that put you out of commission for a week.

When you have roommates who stay up later than you or have kids over until all hours of the night, getting a quality night's sleep is tough. These issues can be resolved with a little negotiation. Don't be afraid to establish some agreements with your roommates, outlining quiet hours. Also, consider bunking up with those who have similar hours for beauty sleep you do!

You might be surprised at the benefits of good sleep and the dangers of poor sleep! According to the Noran Clinic Sleep Center in Minneapolis, healthy sleep helps to achieve the following:[9]

- Strengthens the immune system
- Heals and rejuvenates the body
- Recharges the mind
- Benefits physical activity

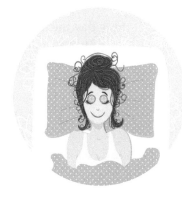

- Improves learning and memory
- Aids sociability
- Fosters good emotional health and happiness
- Improves job functioning

The following list from Noran Clinic Sleep Center details the dangers of inadequate sleep:

- Contributes to cardiovascular problems
- Contributes to neurological problems
- Increases risk of stroke
- Increases risk of anxiety and depression
- Increases risk of obesity and diabetes
- Increases irritability and unhappiness
- Erodes work performance
- Strains personal relationships
- Increases work-related accidents
- Increases automobile accidents
- Reduces libido

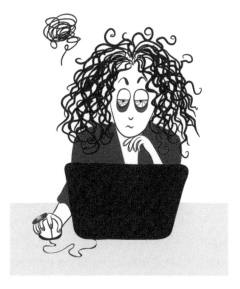

Can't get to sleep? A regular sleep schedule really helps. Try going to bed around the same time every night. Keep in mind that any stimulants or alcohol will probably mess with your ability to sleep. If you are a coffee drinker and have trouble sleeping, stick to less than two cups of coffee (about 200 milligrams of caffeine) a day, and keep away from the Java in the afternoon.

Coffee is not your thing? Remember that energy drinks, tea, soft drinks, chocolate and medicines (including common pain relievers) contain caffeine. Like to party? Yes, alcohol may help you fall asleep, but you probably won't stay asleep because alcohol interrupts regular sleep

I can't count how many times my kids have come home from school and asked, "Does my face look fat?" Guess what? Their faces did look fat! I call it the party puff-face. However, this condition was nothing that a couple of weeks of healthy living didn't cure. Eating well will keep us healthier, help us feel better physically and mentally, and—not that you care—look better!

Eating a poor diet can make us feel physically awful. It can also decrease our energy, which makes combating stress a real challenge. It takes a lot of energy to be productive and face heavy loads of college multi-tasking! In addition, when we fall into bad eating habits, we gain weight and don't feel good about how we look, which adds to our stress.

Last year I received a letter from a young woman named Maddie. This letter tells a story that is not uncommon, but preventable:

> *Dear Susan,*
>
> *I've gained nearly 30 pounds since my freshman year, and twice in the past six months people have asked me if I am pregnant. I don't even enjoy shopping anymore, and I have donated tons of clothes to charities within just the last few months because they no longer fit and make me feel down about myself. When I last saw my doctor, she told me that I am "clinically overweight," which was a huge wake-up call for me.*
>
> *I am going to try my hardest to make life changes this year. I am starting yoga, I joined a gym, and I am trying to eat my healthiest. My goal is to feel more comfortable and confident by my cousin's wedding in April. I've tried losing weight before, and when it doesn't work I get frustrated and discouraged. This time I want to do everything in my power to change.*
>
> *I know my weight gain is primarily due to my diet: I eat out a lot. Fast food is a guilty pleasure and, because I often go right from class to work, I eat quick meals instead of making healthy choices. I also have not been consistent with a workout plan. When I get busy or stressed, I often turn to food rather than the gym. Can you help me?*
>
> *Maddie*

Maddie is one of many young women who has asked me for help during the time between her senior year in high school and senior year in college. This is a time in life when a significant

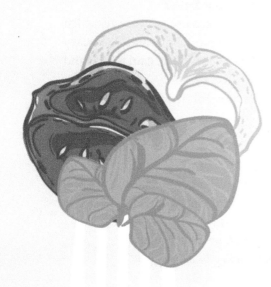

physical transition takes place: young women begin to fill out and get their adult bodies. The combination of nature and bad habits can result in weight gain.

Although many high schools have health and fitness classes, many young people still aren't clear about what is hurting and helping their bodies the most. When they enter college, so many lifestyle changes, stresses and pressures hit them all at once that it's sometimes difficult for them to cope. When I met Maddie, she was a spunky, adorable freshman. A former athlete, she was a healthy weight and never had a care in the world. She ate whatever she wanted and never gave food a second thought. She was active everyday, and her metabolism was not an issue.

Just three years later, she had gained 30 pounds, was depressed and anxious, and didn't know where to turn. A few days after writing her letter to me, she realized she had hit rock bottom physically and mentally and called me in desperation. Climbing out of this deep hole seemed utterly impossible to her. As she wept on the phone, my heart broke for her. She said, "I gained 10 pounds a year: I can't believe I let that happen!" After talking to her about a few details of her daily life, I realized she had no idea how to eat well.

Maddie was a driven, intelligent student who, like a large majority of people, didn't have a very good "how to treat my body well" education. The good news is that Maddie was able to make many changes. She limited her fast food, stopped drinking soda, stopped eating late at night, reduced portion sizes, avoided high-fat foods, and lost nearly 30 pounds in four months. Just by eating a fairly good diet that was far from perfect, she transformed her life! Say "no" to diets and "yes" to reducing bad habits and creating good ones!

Parents have a huge impact on their kids' eating habits, as well. You tend to repeat the behavior you were brought up with. It's total comfort! If mom drinks Coke all day, then it must be OK, right? If you are feeling sad as a kid and mom feeds you sweets, you are most likely to turn to sweets as an adult. Basic education is key. If you didn't get it from your parents, you probably didn't get it.

We are bombarded with nutritional information in the media daily, but face it: most high school and college kids are focused on school, friends, activities and social media. Until your clothes don't fit, you realize your face has blown up like a balloon, or someone asks if you are pregnant, nutrition is not something you pay much attention to.

Do you really know how to make good food choices?

Healthy eating involves much more than you may think. First, we have to know the difference between healthy choices and not-so-healthy choices and how much of each macronutrient we need. Second, we have to do some self-analysis to determine why we eat certain things and when. Third, we have to find the willpower and motivation to select the good choices over the bad. Let's go over the basics and talk about the macronutrients—protein, carbohydrates and fats.

#healthyeating

Protein

Proteins contain four calories per gram and serve many important functions in the body. They are responsible for the forming of the brain, nervous system, blood, muscle, skin and hair. They are also responsible for transporting iron, vitamins, minerals, fats and oxygen.

For some, getting enough protein is a challenge, but it's a key component of weight loss. You burn more calories processing protein, and it takes longer to leave your stomach, so it keeps you satiated. When it comes to resistance training, getting enough protein is especially important because protein is responsible for building lean muscle, which not only makes you stronger and more toned, but fires up your metabolism.

Best choices for protein include:

- Low-fat milk and cheese products
- Eggs
- Lean meats
- Fish
- Nuts
- Legumes

If you have trouble getting enough protein or eating some of these foods, you can mix some good protein powders in a shake for a great protein supplement.

Carbohydrates

Carbohydrates contain about four calories per gram and are a key source of energy. Carbohydrates are found in bread, pasta, potatoes, fruits and vegetables. Our bodies love the fiber, vitamins and minerals we get from the "good" carbs found in whole grains, fruits and vegetables.

However, try to use portion control with the white starchy carbs like refined white rice and pastas. They have been altered, leaving them with less healthy fiber and natural nutrients. What's so great about fiber? Fiber helps to normalize bowel movements, lowers cholesterol levels, controls blood sugar levels, and last but not least, helps maintain a healthy weight! High-fiber foods help you to stay fuller longer and tend to have fewer calories for the same amount of food. There are whole-grain options that have not been stripped of the healthful bran and germ.

Put the brakes on naughty snack items like chips and crackers, most of which are loaded with fat and sodium. Finally, avoid simple sugars found in colas, juices, candy, muffins and desserts.

Don't worry about the sugars in fruits and vegetables. Sticking to fresh and natural foods is the best way to go. It's the added sugars we need to worry about. Aside from weight gain and other health issues, eating a diet high in sugar and refined flours can put you on a blood-sugar, roller-coaster ride. Energy levels and moods can spike and then plummet, ultimately leaving you down in the dumps. No college student needs that!

Food labels can be very deceiving so be careful and check out the packaging. The following terms are basically synonymous with sugar:

- Maltose
- Sucrose
- High fructose corn syrup
- Molasses
- Cane sugar

- Corn sweetener
- Raw sugar
- Syrup
- Honey
- Fruit juice concentrates

According to the American Heart Association, women should consume no more than 100 calories (6 level teaspoons) of added sugar a day, and men should limit their sugar to 150 calories (8 level teaspoons) a day.[10]

Each gram of sugar contains four calories, so if you see a label that says 15 grams of sugar, that equals 60 calories. Four grams of sugar equals one teaspoon of granulated sugar.

Be aware! Did you know that:

- An average muffin often packs close to 8 teaspoons of sugar?
- A medium Coke can have over 14 teaspoons of sugar?
- A tablespoon of ketchup contains 1 teaspoon of sugar?
- A can of tomato soup contains close to 4 teaspoons of sugar?
- A 12-ounce glass of orange juice can contain 10 teaspoons of sugar?

So much sugar is hidden in our foods that even the healthiest sounding packaged foods are the worst culprits. Often packaging is marketed with healthy statements like "low fat" or "fat free," but that doesn't mean it's not loaded with sugar!

More about whole grains

Whole grains are an important part of our diet, but when it comes to breads, these labels can be deceiving, too. "Brown" doesn't necessarily mean "good"! Find labels that say "whole wheat," "100% whole wheat" or "whole grain rye." Look at the labels, and try to buy breads that list "whole grain" as the first ingredient.

Watch out for refined grains like "unbleached enriched wheat flour," "multigrain," "wheat flour," or "100% wheat." "Multigrain" means different kinds of grains, which could be entirely refined. During the process of refining, many beneficial nutrients, including fiber, vitamins and minerals, are removed, leaving a product that has a longer shelf life. If your label claims 2.5 grams or more of fiber per serving, you are good to go! Whole is the magic word when it comes to bread!

Fats

Fats contain about nine calories per gram and should be limited to 20 to 35 percent of your daily food intake. Dietary fat is necessary because it plays a role in insulating cell structure, nerve transmission, vitamin absorption and hormone production. Not all fats are created equal, however. It's important to have some knowledge about the various types of fats because they have different effects on your body. The four types of fat are saturated, trans, polyunsaturated and monounsaturated fats.

According to The American Heart Association, saturated fats should be limited to no more than 7 percent of your daily food intake per day. Saturated fats are primarily found in animal food sources like fatty beef, lamb, pork, poultry with skin, cream, cheese, whole and 2 percent fat milk, in addition to baked goods and fried foods.

You probably have noticed manufacturers touting the fact that they have "0 trans fats" on their labels. This tells you that trans fats are dangerous, and these food companies want you to know they are listening and trying to do something about it. Most trans fats are created during a process that adds hydrogen to liquid vegetable oils to make them more solid. The process of hydrogenation is used to enhance flavor and texture and prolong shelf life. The American Heart Association recommends that you consume no more than 1 percent of your daily food intake from trans fats.

Trans fats are still found in many processed foods, including margarine, snack items, frozen foods and premixed products. Also, be aware of the term "partially hydrogenated." Oils that are partially hydrogenated are trans fats. A label may say the product contains zero trans fats if the trans fat content is less than .5 grams per serving. However, they must list "partially hydrogenated vegetable oil" if that is an ingredient in the item.

Both trans and saturated fats raise our bad cholesterol (LDL), which can lead to heart disease. However, trans fats also lower our good cholesterol (HDL), which is a double whammy!

Mono- or polyunsaturated fats are much better for you than saturated and trans fats. They are found primarily in vegetable oils and foods containing vegetable oils. Studies have shown that these unsaturated fats improve blood cholesterol levels, decreasing risk of heart disease.

All this information helps us to understand the butter-versus-margarine debate. Butter has gotten a bad wrap because it's high in saturated fat and cholesterol. Margarine, on the other hand, is made with vegetable oils that are not saturated fats. The problem is that not all margarines are alike; some of the solid stick brands contain trans fats and other chemicals.

Experts at the Mayo Clinic suggest using trans-fat-free tub spreads or, better yet, eliminate the spreads completely, especially for those watching their heart health. Others feel that butter, made from natural cream, is best because it does not contain additives. Regardless, using a small amount of any spread is the way to go!

Below is a list of unsaturated fat options. Read labels and make good fat choices that can have positive effects on your heart health and weight.

Basic "good" fat sources are:

- Fish
- Nuts
- Avocados and guacamole
- Olives
- Peanut butter (preferably natural)
- Almond butter
- Dark chocolate (woo hoo!)
- Canola oil
- Olive oil

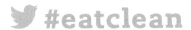 # #eatclean

Don't forget Omega-3 fatty acids

Omega-3 fatty acids are polyunsaturated fatty acids that are required for many functions of human health but are not produced in the body, which makes it imperative to get them through our diet. Omega-3 fatty acids are known to reduce inflammation and the risk of heart disease. Research shows that these fatty acids aid in brain function, helping us to focus, concentrate and ease symptoms of depression and dementia.

Some excellent sources of Omega-3 fatty acids are:

- Fatty fish: salmon, herring, mackerel, lake trout, tuna, sardines and anchovies (The American Heart Association recommends at least two servings a week of fish.)
- Vegetable oils: soybean, flaxseed, olive and canola oil
- Green vegetables: spinach, kale, Brussels sprouts and edamame
- Walnuts
- Flaxseed

Sprinkle some flaxseed on your cereal, cook and spread with olive or canola oil, mix walnuts in your oatmeal, and try to get fish and green vegetables in your diet: you might notice you have a better brain!

Warning: avoid processed foods

The best way to reduce sugar, sodium, preservatives and bad fats in your diet is to avoid processed foods. Processed foods are engineered to have a long shelf life and taste good, no matter what the consequences! The ingredient list is often a mile long, and many of the words you can't pronounce. These foods are commonly loaded with fat and sodium.

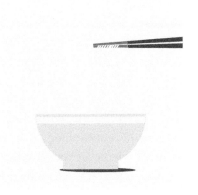

Avoiding process foods can be difficult in college, but being aware and eating fresh foods when possible will make a huge difference in your life. Do you and your friends feast on ramen noodles and easy mac? For 25 cents a package, who wouldn't? Maybe it's not a bad idea to have these quick packaged meals on hand for emergencies or a once-in-a-while pasta/salt craving. But please don't make these your main staple, because you may just blow up like a puffer fish from all the sodium!

Here are the most common types of processed foods:

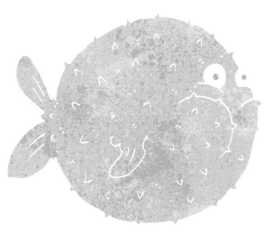

- Canned foods
- Breads and pastas made with refined white flour instead of whole grains
- Packaged snack foods such as chips and candies
- Frozen dinners
- Packaged cakes and cookies
- Boxed meal mixes
- Sugary breakfast cereals
- Processed meats

Sodium

What's so bad about sodium? Many people don't care about the warnings regarding excess sodium because it really doesn't make you fat with calories. However, it might make you look a little swollen! Excess sodium builds up in your blood and holds onto water. This water retention creates more work for your heart, causing high blood pressure, which in turn can lead to heart and kidney disease, stroke and congestive heart failure.

Dietary guidelines recommend limiting sodium to less than 2300 milligrams a day for healthy young adults.

Here are just a few examples of food items loaded with sodium:

- 1 serving (1/2 cup) condensed chicken noodle soup = 890 milligrams of sodium
- One tablespoon of soy sauce = 1000 milligrams of sodium
- Two slices of processed sandwich deli ham = 730 milligrams of sodium

It's impossible for most people to avoid processed foods completely. Often your busy college life will require foods that are convenient. However, awareness is the key. Eating natural, fresh foods whenever you have the opportunity will be worth it in the long run for both your health and your appearance. A canned vegetable is better than no vegetables and gives you some nutrients you won't get in a bag of chips. It's about weighing the disadvantages against the advantages and making the best choices you can with what is available to you.

Buy as many items as you can from the perimeters of the grocery store, where you will find most of the natural, whole foods. The center aisles are filled with processed foods that don't have to be refrigerated.

If you have the opportunity to get a fast-food burger high in fat and sodium or a sandwich made with fresh lean meat, veggies and whole-grain bread, I hope you will take the latter option. If you have analyzed your daily food intake and realize you haven't had a vegetable yet, maybe you will get that side salad with your dinner. It's all about awareness and education about nutrition.

Nutrition affects your entire body, including your brain. Do the best you can without being hard on yourself. This is the start to creating good habits and thoughtful eating, even though the circumstances of college life don't make it easy. Be proud of your intention and your efforts to be good to your body.

The United States Department of Agriculture (USDA) guidelines recommend that healthy adults consume the following percentages of macronutrients:[11]

- Carbohydrates: 45 to 65 percent (Whole grains, fruits and veggies are the best!)
- Protein: 10 to 35 percent (Keep it lean if you can!)
- Fat: 20 to 35 percent (Remember the "good" fats!)

Here's the healthiest way to fill your plate.

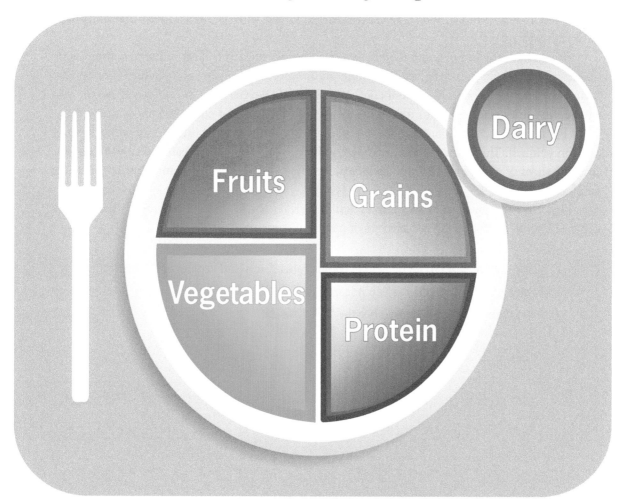

Calcium

Calcium is important for bone health not only during childhood, but at every age. Bone mass peaks between the ages of 14 and 24. After our twenties, bone density gradually decreases, which can cause significant health problems. The amount of bone mass a young woman has when she is 35 will be a strong determinant for her risk of osteoporosis later in life. Osteoporosis for men is a very real problem, as well. Women see bone loss earlier due to menopausal changes. However, both men and women are affected equally later in life.

I worked with a lovely woman in her seventies who had osteoporosis. Her back was hunched, and she was so very frail that I feared even the slightest misstep could cause a major fracture. All of us want to be rockin' when we are 70, not fragile. If you pay attention to your calcium intake and participate in weight-bearing exercise, you will have a better chance at maintaining your bone density.

Adults ages 19 to 50 should get 1000 milligrams of calcium per day, preferably through food and beverages.[12]

Great sources of calcium-rich, low-fat foods include dairy products such as:

- Low-fat milk
- Low-fat yogurt
- Low-fat cheese (Swiss, low-fat mozzarella, cottage and feta are good choices.)

Avoid dairy products that have the word "whole" in the label like "whole milk product." Whole in the dairy world tends to mean more fat. Items labeled "fat free" often contain excess sugar and other unnatural chemicals. Go with the "low fat" label!

Some non-dairy options include:

- Lactose-free dairy products
- Calcium fortified foods and beverages such as cereal and orange juice
- Oatmeal
- Salmon
- Tuna
- Kale
- Spinach

Vitamin D

Vitamin D is imperative because it assists our bodies with calcium absorption. Adults ages 19-50 should get 600 international units of vitamin D.[13] Our bodies are able to produce vitamin D rather quickly with sun exposure. You can get smaller amounts of vitamin D through some of the following foods and beverages:

- Fatty fish like salmon
- Canned tuna
- Fortified milk

- Fortified cereal
- Egg yolks

If you are unable to get enough calcium through your diet or if you feel you could be vitamin D deficient due to lack of sun exposure, it's important to speak with your doctor to find out if you are a candidate for supplementation and how much is safe to take.

For more information on nutrition guidelines, health tips, food tracking, sample menus and recipes, go to choosemyplate.gov

Water

Water makes up 50 to 70 percent of the human body, making it the body's largest component. Water protects vital organs, regulates body temperature, and aids in nutrient absorption and all biochemical reactions. It is imperative that we stay hydrated. A 10 percent loss of water can cause serious problems. Dehydration can lead to fatigue and make you feel really crummy! According to Weill Cornell Medical College, some studies suggest that even mild dehydration can slow your metabolism and decrease your energy.[14]

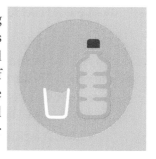

Experts recommend consuming 64 ounces (eight 8-ounce glasses) of water throughout the day. However, everyone has variable daily activity, so it's most important to listen to our bodies and let thirst be the guide. Better yet, stay ahead of it if you can! Also, be aware that caffeine and alcohol are dehydrating: we need to drink extra water when we are having a latte or a beer. To be healthy, we need to be hydrated because our body's functions depend upon it.[15] If you look at your pee and it's really yellow, you better grab a big glass of water or two!

Weight loss coaches often recommend drinking a big glass of water before meals to curb the appetite. If you tend to overeat, this might help you control your portions and hydrate yourself at the same time!

Do's and don'ts in restaurants and cafeterias

What do we think of when we hear the word "college" combined with "eating"? A pizza frenzy feed at two o'clock in the morning, right? Let's eat half a pizza and go to bed! Listen, my friend, you cannot justify pizza because it has protein and a little bit of tomato sauce and, if you are lucky, some peppers and mushrooms!

Let's talk about pizza. White dough (bad carb!), gobs of cheese, pepperoni and sausage (major fat!)—and how many college kids have vegetables on their pizza? And, at two in the morning, do you stick to one serving? Not! One serving of pizza is one slice, and that's like eating one potato chip. Who does that? Large portions are one of the main reasons for obesity in our society. A three-ounce serving of meat is the size of a deck of cards or your fist. The average serving sizes in restaurants may be three to four times what we actually need!

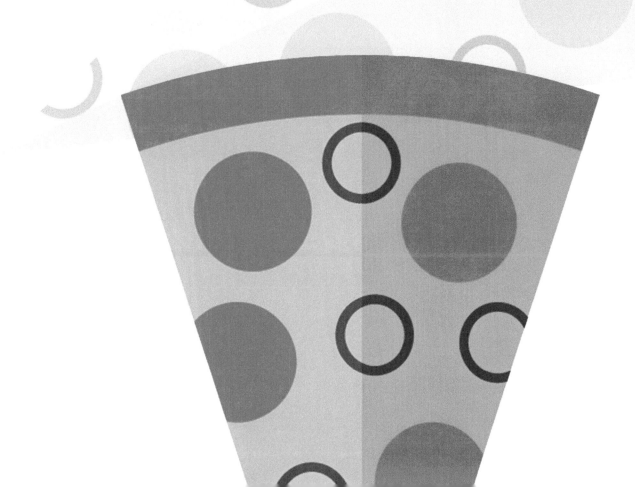

Important tip

Keep in mind that restaurants are rated by flavor, and flavor is often created with fat and sugar. The bad news is that few of us know what size a healthy serving is! One way to control portion size at a restaurant is to ask for a "to go" box right away and put half of your meal in the container before you take your first bite. What's not to love about having yummy leftovers at school? Also, ask for the dressings and sauces to be served on the side. That way you can control how "lite" you want to keep your meal.

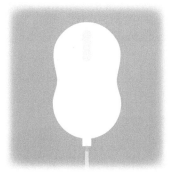

A computer mouse = 3 ounces of meat or a half cup of rice or pasta

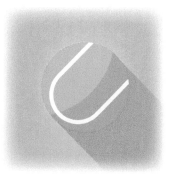

A baseball or tennis ball = 1 serving of fruit

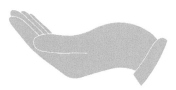

1 handful = 1 ounce of nuts or small candies

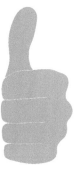

Thumb = 1 ounce of cheese
Tip of the thumb from the knuckle up = 1 teaspoon of butter or mayo
3 teaspoons = 1 tablespoon

Breakfast choices

When it comes to breakfast, try not to skip it. Breakfast recharges the body and the brain and allows you to function more efficiently in every way! Skipping breakfast has been linked to weight gain and obesity. Often, people who skip breakfast tend to overeat later in the day and snack on unhealthy foods.

Here are a few tips for a healthy breakfast:

- Stay away from fatty breakfast meats like bacon and sausage.
- Combine yogurt and fruit sprinkled with a few walnuts, natural granola or a whole-grain cereal.
- Enjoy whole-grain toast with limited spreads.
- Combine whole-grain cereals with natural fruit.
- Have a bowl of plain oatmeal with fresh fruit or limited sweetener.
- Add veggies like cooked spinach, mushrooms and peppers to your eggs.

Eggs are a good source of protein, and the yolks do contain healthy vitamins and minerals. However, they are high in cholesterol. Sometimes you might consider ordering an omelet prepared with egg whites or make scrambled eggs using one yolk and a few egg whites. Some nutritionists suggest limiting egg yolks to four per week, and some say one a day is a healthy guideline. Regardless, be aware that consuming egg yolks in moderation is OK for most healthy individuals!

Subs and sandwiches

- Choose a 6-inch rather than a 12-inch sub.
- Choose whole-grain bread or take the top off your sandwich and eat it open-faced.
- Choose lean meats like chicken or turkey.
- Limit yourself to one or two slices of lower-fat cheese (Swiss or mozzarella).
- Add as many veggies as you want.
- Choose a low-fat dressing or mustard instead of mayo. Italian dressing is a great choice.

Pizza and Italian foods

- Choose thin-crust pizza.
- Ask for half the cheese.

- Avoid high-calorie, fattening meats like pepperoni and sausage.
- Include veggies.

Pasta

- Order dishes with veggies and seafood or chicken rather than heavy sausage entrees.
- Avoid cream or butter-based sauces and order tomato-based red sauces or a little olive oil.
- Eat plain rolls or breadsticks in place of cheesy or butter-laden breads.
- Italian portions can be huge, so take half of it home.

Burgers

- Stick to grilled chicken instead of fried.
- Order single-patty hamburgers.
- Go for the side salad or baked potato rather than fries.
- Limit or avoid mayo and cream-based dressings or toppings.
- If you need that French fry fix, split a small order with your friend.

Mexican food

- Go for the grilled meat items.
- Choose a soft taco or "bowl."
- Pick black beans rather than refried beans.
- Say "yes" to veggies.
- Limit sour cream and cheese.

Asian food

- Select broth-based soups.
- Go for entrees that are stir-fried, broiled, steamed or roasted.
- Stay away from battered or deep-fried entrees.
- Include lots of veggies.
- Choose steamed brown rice rather than fried rice. (So sorry.)
- Use portion control with Asian food because it's easy to overdo when servings are large.

Popular food chains and some healthy food options

It's hard to avoid fast food when you are a college student and always on the run. But do what you can to eat fresh foods and limit the visits to fast-food restaurants. It can be more dangerous to your health than you think. The excessive sodium and fat tastes good, but a lot of it can be deadly—aside from the fact you might double your waistline!

The good news is that fast-food restaurants are offering more healthy options all the time. Some chains, like Panera®, Chipotle® and Noodles®, offer mostly fresh ingredients. Study the options below, and try to make the best choices most of the time!

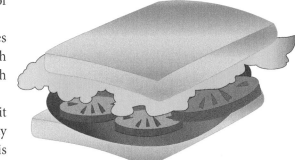

Remember that some burgers and sandwiches contain 800 to 1200 calories and are overloaded with dangerous salt and fat! A 40-ounce soda or fruit punch contains more than 500 calories!

We want to get the biggest bang for our buck when it comes to combining macronutrients. A cheese chilito may have the same calorie content as a soft taco, but the taco is bigger and includes the veggie nutrients your body needs. A pile of cheese in a cheese chilito may have some calcium, but it is loaded with fat. A little cheese can be healthful, but don't go overboard! Below are some tips for eating at some of the popular fast-food restaurant chains. Some of the options will change periodically, so if you have a favorite or convenient fast food restaurant you frequent, take the time to look up its nutrition chart online.

Arby's®

The plain Roast Beef Classic sandwich, Roast Turkey and Swiss Wrap and Roast Turkey Farmhouse Salad with Light Italian or Balsamic Vinaigrette dressing are my picks at Arby's.

Burger King®

If you are looking for a healthful snack or breakfast, try the Fruit Topped Maple Flavored Quaker Oatmeal or a Fruit Smoothie. If you are craving a burger, the Hamburger, Whopper Jr. or Veggie Burger without mayo are your best options. The Tendergrill Chicken Sandwich without mayo keeps your intake under 400 calories, as well. Add a side salad or the Fresh Apple Fries, and you have a full meal. The Chicken, Apple & Cranberry Garden Wrap or Salad and the Tendergrill Chicken Garden Salad with low-fat or fat-free dressing are meals with nutritious ingredients.

Chipotle®

Chipotle is one of the few fast-food restaurants that offer many options for fresh food. The portions are very large, however. The tortilla alone packs on 290 calories! If you are watching calories, you might lose the tortilla and have a burrito bowl or salad instead. Go easy on the rice, choose chicken or steak, include the veggies, and avoid sour cream and cheese. The guacamole is higher in calories, but it contains "good" fat, so using it as a dressing in moderation beats the sour cream!

Chick-Fil-A®

The Yogurt Parfait with Granola and Oatmeal with Toppings offer some good nutrition for a snack or breakfast. The Chik-n-minis are actually one of the better breakfast sandwiches available at fast-food restaurants. For lunch or dinner, the Chargrilled Chicken Cool Wrap, the Chargrilled Chicken Sandwich and the Grilled Market Salad with Reduced Fat Berry Balsamic Vinaigrette Dressing are among the healthier options.

Jack in the Box®

Jack's Real Fruit Smoothies are great, fat-free breakfast and snack options. Healthy lunches and dinners include Grilled Chicken Salad, Chicken Teriyaki Bowl, Grilled Chicken Strips with Teriyaki Dipping Sauce and Chicken Fajita Pita.

KFC®

Grilled chicken is a tasty and healthy option at KFC if you strip the skin. Order green beans or corn for a side. If you love mashed potatoes and gravy, dip your fork in a side of gravy rather than dumping a boatload on your potatoes.

McDonald's®

The Fruit & Maple Oatmeal and the Fruit 'N Yogurt Parfait are healthful options for a breakfast or snack. If you are craving a breakfast sandwich, choose the McDonald's Egg McMuffin: it has more protein and fiber than many of its competitors. The Grilled Chicken Classic Sandwich, Grilled Honey Mustard Snack Wrap and Caesar Salad with Grilled Chicken and light dressing are some of the better McDonald's options. Don't be afraid to order a Hamburger and Apple Dipper Happy Meal if you're not a kid. It's not a bad choice no matter how big you are!

Panera Bread®

The Mediterranean Egg White on Ciabatta is my breakfast sandwich choice. The Smoked Turkey Breast Sandwich, Mediterranean Veggie Sandwich, and Tuna Salad Sandwich are safe bets for lunch, but just go with half a sandwich and get a cup of healthy soup or a half salad on their "you pick two" menu. Order any of Panera's light or reduced sugar or reduced fat dressings on your salads. Thai Chicken Salad, Spinach Power Salad, Asian Sesame Chicken Salad and Fugi Apple Chicken Salad all offer good nutrition! To avoid cream-based soups, try ordering Low Fat Chicken Noodle Soup, Low Fat Chicken Tortilla Soup with Tortilla Strips, Low Fat Vegetarian Black Bean Soup or Low Fat Vegetarian Garden Vegetable Soup. Do not order them in a bread bowl (560 calories) if you will be tempted to eat the whole thing!

Subway®

Subway offers a variety of egg white, flatbread breakfast sandwiches that contain less than 200 calories. My picks would be the Egg White & Cheese and the Egg White with Cheese and Avocado. For lunch you can't go wrong with a six-inch sub on nine-grain wheat bread, with lean meat and loaded with fresh veggies. The Veggie Delite, Oven Roasted Chicken, Turkey Breast and Roast Beef Sandwiches are good choices.

Subway has good soup and salad options, as well. Vegetable Beef Soup, Minestrone and Chicken Noodle Soup contain much less fat than some of the cream-based varieties. However, soup often has a high sodium content. You can make an even more healthful meal by losing the bread and having all the ingredients in a chopped salad. Lower calorie toppings at Subway include Fat Free Honey Mustard, Fat Free Sweet Onion, mustard, light mayo, olive oil and vinegar. Remember to ask your server to go light on the dressing. If you don't, your sandwich or salad may be swimming in fat and contain many more calories than you think!

Taco Bell®

The Fresco Menu has replaced high-fat cheeses and sauces with a healthful pico de gallo fresh salsa, keeping these items to less than 350 calories! My picks would be the Fresco Soft Tacos (under 200 cals)! Better yet, you can take one of the higher calorie items and turn it into a Fresco by asking them to replace the usual fattening sauces with the restaurant's flavorful, low-cal pico de gallo salsa. If that's not your thing, go for a regular Chicken or Beef Soft Taco. My pick for a side is Black Beans or Black Beans with Rice.

Wendy's®

Wendy's Chili or a Broccoli Cheese Potato can be a satisfying snack or, if paired with a side salad, eaten as a meal. If you are in the mood for a burger, stick with the Jr. Hamburger or Jr. Cheeseburger. My favorite sandwich choice is the Ultimate Chicken Grill.

Ideas for refrigerated snacks in your dorm room

Healthful items that you might have room to keep in a small, dorm fridge are:

- Skim milk
- Low-fat yogurt
- Low-fat cottage cheese
- String mozzerella cheese
- Baby carrots
- Hummus

Foods that don't have to be refrigerated

Healthful foods you could keep in your dorm room that don't need refrigeration are:[16]

- Fruits such as apples, oranges and bananas
- Dried fruit, but keep in mind there is added sugar
- Whole-grain bread or bagel thins
- Whole-grain crackers
- Nuts
- A jar of natural peanut butter
- Mini cans of water-packed tuna
- Microwavable containers of low-fat soup
- Low-fat, microwavable popcorn
- Oatmeal packets
- Whole-grain cereals
- Protein bars (preferably that contain at least 10 grams of protein and 3 grams of fiber per serving and no more than 15 grams of sugar or 5 grams of fat)
- Cereal bars that contain 3 grams of fiber if possible

Keep some of the above items in your car or backpack so when you're starving before or after class you have a go-to item that isn't full of fat and sugar!

Hold the soda and the fruit juice!

Soda can be a really naughty thing! One 32-ounce Big Gulp® of regular cola contains about 400 calories of sugar topped off with large amounts of sodium!

Fruit juice sounds healthy and, unlike soda, does contain some nutrients, but you are better off eating an orange (80 calories of natural, filling fiber) than chugging a glass of juice (up to 140 calories in 10 ounces). Try spiking a small amount of fruit juice with sparkling water—oh, so refreshing!

Energy drinks like Gatorade® also contain a lot of sugar. Stick to water as much as possible, and add a slice of lemon. Or try some unsweetened ice tea. Finally, watch the special coffees that are laden with creams and sugar.

Coffee

Lately we have been hearing about the benefits of coffee. Coffee has disease-fighting antioxidants, but it's still important to realize that too much caffeine can have adverse affects on your health. Make sure to listen to your body for signs of too much caffeine. Over-stimulating your body can lead to higher stress levels and energy crashes. If you notice you are getting the jitters, headaches, heart palpitations, insomnia, shaking, trembling or stomach irritation, cut your intake of caffeine. If you have gastrointestinal issues or heart problems, you may have medical reasons to abstain from coffee.

In addition, be aware of all the added calories that come with the endless, tasty options that include chocolate, caramel, syrups, sugars and creams. All those extra yummy additions add up, especially if you drink them everyday. Did you know that Caribou®'s Berry White Mocha Cooler contains 670 calories? The company's Mint Condition Mocha Cooler contains 700 calories! That is 100 to 150 calories more than a Big Mac at McDonalds®! Do some calorie-counting research if you love the specialty coffees, and if you want to be really good, use a little bit of skim milk in your black coffee!

Also, beware of bottles of sweetened tea because the sugar content can be very high. Be leery of unnatural energy boosters like caffeine pills and over-the-top caffeinated beverages. They might help you get through an all-night study session, but eventually you will crash, resulting in more stress and possibly sickness and addiction.

Alcohol

It might seem like a good idea to have a few drinks after a hard day: life feels good for a short time, but the unresolved stress will just come raging back. We will talk more about the risks of alcohol in Chapter 8, but from a nutritional standpoint, alcohol contains seven calories per gram, and those calories are empty calories: alcohol has absolutely no nutritional value.

I don't want to be a downer, but there is a direct correlation between alcohol and a larger waistline, and it's not just the extra calories. If your liver is too busy burning off alcohol, it can't burn off fat. Also, alcohol affects the hormones that regulated our sense of satiety and so can cause overeating. Moderate consumption of alcohol does have some health benefits. However, listen up: moderate consumption means **one drink a day for women** and **two drinks a day for men**, not a bottle or a 12-pack!

Binge drinking is common in college, so keep in mind that excess alcohol consumption can lead to cirrhosis of the liver. Also, many medications are dangerous when combined with alcohol, so be aware of that! And ladies, if you think you could be pregnant, stay away from the bottle! Alcohol can cause birth defects.

How to avoid the "beer belly" if you choose to drink alcohol:

- Stick to "light" beer.
- Use mixers like club soda, diet tonic, limes and lemons instead of regular colas and high-calorie juices.
- Spike your white wine with club soda—half the calories, half the headache.
- Tell yourself how many beverages you will allow yourself before you walk into the party, or better yet, bring only the amount you plan on drinking, and you will be more likely to use good judgment.
- Water, water, water.
- And—yes—what about "shots" of alcohol? They are dangerous, and I don't recommend them! Don't be hard on your liver by overloading it with alcohol. Dilute it with a low or no-cal mixer.

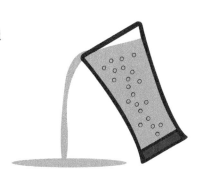

Supplements

Nutritional supplements include vitamins, minerals, herbs, meal supplements, sports nutrition products, natural food supplements, and other products used to boost the nutritional content of the diet. Many products out there claim to promote weight loss, better athletic performance, better sleep, and more energy. Although many supplements do have health benefits, they are not all regulated by the FDA, so one must use caution when taking them.

I always tell my clients to discuss the use of any supplement with their primary physicians. Many supplements do have risks associated with them, and some should not be combined with other medications or used in the presence of certain health conditions.

Keep in mind that there is not a magic pill that will make weight loss an easy task, at least without risk. Getting your nutrients through real, healthful food is the healthiest way. When it comes to your body shortcuts are not the answer.

If you have questions about commonly used supplements and herbs, go to the National Institutes of Health Office of Dietary Supplements, http://www.dietary-supplements.info.nih.gov/factsheets/list-all/MVMs/

Have you moved out of the dorms?
Now you can make some healthful meals!

Refuel your brain and body with breakfast

You have probably heard that breakfast is the most important meal of the day. As I mentioned earlier, this is especially true if you are a college student! When you are hungry and low on energy, concentrating on anything is really difficult! Food is fuel for the brain. If you eat a healthy breakfast at your place, you might avoid high caloric snacks from vending machines or late-in-the-day binges on whatever you can find!

Satisfy yourself with smoothies

Smoothies are a great way to get a head start on your fruits and vegetables each day. Don't be afraid to create your own smoothie combinations. You can add any fruit and a variety of vegetables to your morning blend. Try some of the recipes below to get you started, and soon you will become a pro at smoothie making!

Basics ingredients to keep on hand for smoothies:

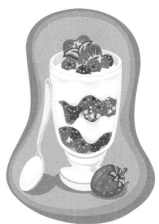

- Frozen strawberries or raspberries
- Frozen blueberries
- Bananas
- Yogurt
- Peanut butter
- Milk
- A sweetener like honey or agave nectar
- Spinach or kale

Peanut butter and banana smoothie.
Blend the following ingredients:

    10 ounces skim milk

    1 tablespoon peanut butter

    1 medium banana

    6 ice cubes

Strawberry banana smoothie.
Blend the following ingredients:

    ½ banana

    ½ cup frozen strawberries

    1 ½ cups milk

Greek yogurt and fruit smoothie.
Blend the following ingredients:

    6 ounces blueberry Greek yogurt

    1 banana

    4 frozen strawberries

    ¼ cup cold water or milk

    4 ice cubes

Blueberry, spinach and banana smoothie with extra protein.
Blend the following ingredients:

    2/3 cup plain Greek yogurt

    1 banana

    1 cup frozen blueberries

    1 cup spinach leaves

    ½ cup milk

    2 teaspoons protein powder (optional)

    1 tablespoon agave nectar or honey

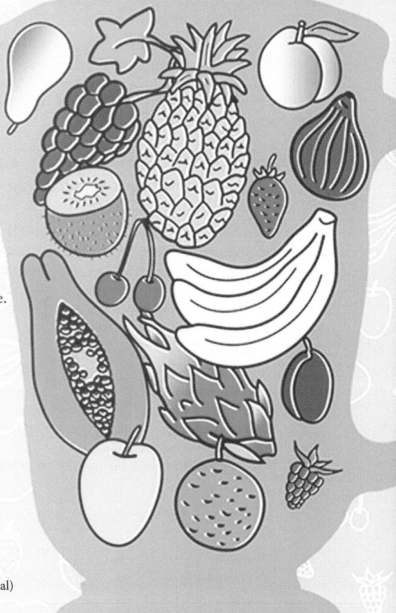

Oatmeal with some yummy additions

Oatmeal is convenient, healthful and great for weight control. The soluble fiber helps to slow down the digestive process, which keeps you feeling fuller longer. Oatmeal is packed with vitamins, minerals and antioxidants and is a good source of fiber and protein. Steel-cut oats are the least processed, but plain instant oatmeal is a great option for people on the go. Add some flavor with fresh or frozen fruit, dried fruit, a dollop of jam, chopped nuts or granola.

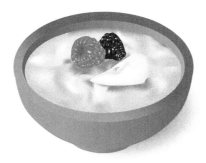

Yogurt

Yogurt is a good source of carbohydrates and protein. Greek yogurt has more protein than regular yogurt and will keep you satiated longer. However, be aware of the high sugar content many brands contain. Opt for a plain yogurt and add fruit, granola, crunchy cereal, mixed nuts or walnuts for additional flavor and crunch.

Whole-grain toast with peanut butter and banana

Spread some peanut butter on whole-grain bread and then slice a banana on top. (If you want to be really healthy, use natural peanut butter.) Here you have your whole grain, fruit, protein and "good" fat all in one delicious combination!

Eggs

Eggs are a great, natural source of protein. If you are watching your fat intake, you can use more egg whites than yokes. For instance, if you are scrambling eggs, you might use three egg whites and one egg yolk. The fat is in the yoke, but the yoke also contains vitamins, and we do need some fat in our diets. If you want to get some extra nutrients, add veggies such as sautéed

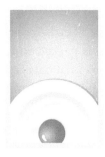

fresh spinach, mushrooms, tomatoes, peppers or onions. If you have vegetables left over from last night's dinner, you can use those, too.

Sauté the vegetables in a little olive oil or butter, then remove them from the pan. Pop a piece of whole-grain bread in the toaster and scramble or cook eggs sunny side up. Layer the vegetables and eggs on the toast, and you have a delicious combo of protein, vitamins, healthy carbohydrates and "good" fat!

Ideas for lunch and dinner

Making a pot of healthy, hearty soup is a great way to have a go-to meal that you can heat up quickly. Soup requires some prep time, but you might try cooking it on a Sunday. Then it will be ready for you at the busy beginning of your week.

Eating a big bowl of vegetable soup daily is a fabulous way to reduce your caloric intake while consuming healthy doses of essential vitamins and minerals.

Basic recipe for a delicious, healthful vegetable soup

    4 teaspoons olive oil
    1 medium onion, diced
    2 medium carrots, diced
    2 celery stalks, diced
    2 medium garlic cloves, finely chopped (or buy a jar of chopped garlic)
    2 medium potatoes, diced
    2 cups additional vegetables (such as red pepper, cabbage or mushrooms)
    1 quart low-sodium chicken or vegetable broth

Heat the olive oil in a large saucepan on medium-high heat. Add the onion and cook, stirring occasionally, until translucent (about 5 minutes). Add the carrots, celery and garlic and cook until the garlic is fragrant (about 2 minutes). Add the potatoes, additional vegetables and broth and bring to a boil. Then reduce the heat to low and simmer until the potatoes can be pierced with a fork (15 to 25 minutes).

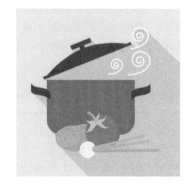

Season the soup with salt and pepper. For extra flavor, add a teaspoon or two of dried parsley flakes, Italian seasoning, or a combination of thyme, oregano and basil. For extra protein, add some rotisserie chicken.

Sandwiches and tortillas

Don't discount the value of quick and easy sandwiches! If they are made with whole-grain bread, lean protein and vegetables, they can help keep you healthy and satisfied. Wraps and quesadillas made with whole-wheat tortillas are also great options and can be heated up in your microwave, as well. The following recipes include cheese, which is an excellent source of calcium and protein but should be consumed in moderation. Try mozzarella or Swiss for a lower fat option. Cheese is optional, however. These are just ideas. Be creative: you will discover many yummy combinations that include healthy nutrients!

Bean, cheese and tomato roll-ups

Spread canned, refried beans or black beans (even healthier) on a whole-wheat tortilla, and sprinkle lightly with cheese. Heat in the microwave for 30 to 45 seconds. Add tomatoes or shredded lettuce or both. Then roll the tortilla up or flip it over in half.

Meat and cheese roll-ups

Place turkey or ham on a whole-wheat tortilla, and sprinkle lightly with cheese. Heat in the microwave for 30 to 45 seconds. Add tomatoes, mushrooms, cucumbers, onions or lettuce. Then roll the tortilla up or flip it over in half.

Quesadillas

Heat a frying pan to a medium-high heat. Spread a whole-wheat tortilla with a little olive oil or butter, place it in the pan with the buttered side facing down, and sprinkle it with cheese. Add any other fillings you like, such as black beans, peppers, cheese, tomatoes, mushrooms or grilled chicken.

Use a spatula to fold the tortilla over so that it looks like half of a pizza. If you want a crispier texture, flip the quesadilla over and heat it briefly. Put the quesadilla on a plate and cut it into triangles with a pizza cutter. Put salsa into a bowl for dipping, or pull back top of quesadilla and spread the salsa on the inside. Enjoy!

Open-faced veggie sandwich

Sauté peppers and mushrooms in olive oil and sprinkle with salt and cracked pepper. (Start with the peppers; they take a little longer.) Throw in pieces of your favorite cheese in the pan (I like swiss or mozzarella) and toss a little. Pile mixture on toasted, fresh, whole-grain bread.

Open-faced tuna melt with veggies

Ingredients for two:

    5 ounces canned tuna

    1.5 tablespoons Hellman's Light mayo

    1.5 tablespoons pickle relish

    Olive oil

    2 whole-grain bread slices

    Whole-grain or spicy brown mustard

    2 slices of mozzarella, Swiss or "light" cheddar cheese.

    Avocado slices (optional)

    Tomato slices

Mix tuna, mayo and relish. Layer bread slices with mustard, tuna mixture, cheese, avocado, tomato, salt and pepper. Heat olive oil and sandwich on medium heat until cheese starts to melt and bread is golden brown.

Fresh green salads with protein

Salads are a great way to incorporate healthy, low-calorie greens and vegetables into our diets. For convenience, use a bottled dressing of your choice, preferably light. Italian is one of the healthiest options. However, if you prefer homemade dressing, you can stir one up easily with balsamic vinegar and oil. Don't forget to add some lean protein to complete your meal!

Vegetables to add to salad greens:

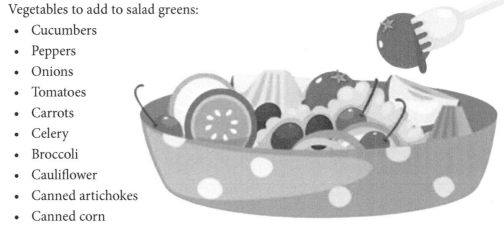

- Cucumbers
- Peppers
- Onions
- Tomatoes
- Carrots
- Celery
- Broccoli
- Cauliflower
- Canned artichokes
- Canned corn
- Any vegetables you have leftover in your fridge, like asparagus or green beans

Great sources of protein for green salads:
- Mozzarella, feta, Swiss or low-fat cottage cheese
- Chicken
- Turkey
- Canned tuna, salmon or crab
- Shrimp
- Hard-boiled eggs
- Canned beans, such as garbanzo, lima or butter beans

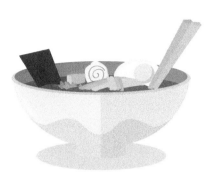

Basic balsamic vinegar and oil dressing

As a general rule, use three parts olive oil to one part vinegar, but you can adjust the proportions to suit your taste. This basic recipe makes one cup:

> ¾ cup extra-virgin olive oil
> ¼ cup balsamic vinegar
> Salt and fresh ground pepper to taste

Pasta salads

Making a big batch of pasta salad is an inexpensive way to create filling, healthy food to keep in your fridge. Red onion, peppers, green or red peppers, broccoli, mushrooms, onion, cucumbers, green or black olives, pine nuts, sunflower seeds, chicken, ham or turkey are all great additions to a pasta salad. Here is a simple pasta salad recipe you might like:

Rainbow pasta salad with tomatoes and cucumbers

Mix cooked rainbow rotini pasta with chopped tomatoes, green onions and cucumbers. Add grated Parmesan cheese and toss with your favorite bottled Italian dressing.

Healthy taco salad

Brown ground turkey and cook with taco seasoning mix according to the directions on the package. Top with lots of shredded lettuce, tomatoes and other healthy options like peppers, black olives, black beans, avocado, and a little shredded cheese. For the crunch, use a corn taco bowl or broken taco chips.

This recipe contains lean protein, fiber, good fat and good carbs. Just go light on the cheese and the shell or chips!

Chicken

Chicken is an excellent source of lean protein. It serves as a great main course or can be added to soup, sandwiches, green salad or pasta salad. The most important thing to remember when preparing chicken is: rinse it and cook it thoroughly! Discard and clean up all drippings from uncooked chicken to prevent any possible bacterial contamination.

Easy, tender baked chicken

Cut a chicken into parts and rub with olive oil. Sprinkle on both sides with salt and freshly ground black pepper. Arrange in pan with the larger pieces in the middle. Bake for 30 minutes at 400 degrees, then lower heat to 350 degrees and bake for another 20 to 30 minutes.

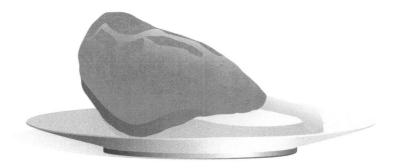

Sautéed chicken

Purchase boneless chicken breasts. Flatten them by placing them between two sheets of plastic wrap and pounding them with some kind of mallet. (This process is completely optional, but it allows for even cooking and creates more tender chicken.)

Sprinkle chicken with salt and pepper, lemon-pepper seasoning, or any other favorite spices. Heat 1 to 2 tablespoons olive oil or canola oil in a skillet over medium heat until hot. Add the chicken, and sauté on both sides for 8 to 12 minutes—until the chicken is slightly browned and no longer pink in the middle. (If you have flattened the chicken, you will need to sauté it for only 6 to 8 minutes.)

Chicken strips or chicken tenders

Cut chicken breasts into strips and prepare according to the directions given above for sautéed chicken. However, reduce the cooking time to just 6 to 8 minutes. Turn the strips occasionally.

Easy baked tilapia or other white fish

    4 tilapia fillets or fillets of any other white fish (for 4 servings)

    2 tablespoons lemon juice

    1 tablespoon butter or margarine, melted

    ½ teaspoon black pepper

    ¼ cup grated Parmesan cheese (optional)

Preheat oven to 375 degrees, and spray a baking sheet with nonstick cooking spray. Rinse fillets under cold water and pat dry. Place the fillets on the baking sheet. Mix lemon juice in melted butter and spread evenly over fish. Sprinkle with black pepper and any other seasoning you wish to use, such as onion powder, garlic powder, dried parsley flakes, dill, basil or oregano. Bake for 30 minutes—until the fillets are completely white and flake apart with a fork. If desired, sprinkle parmesan over fish during the last 5 to 10 minutes of baking time.

If you wish, you can keep individually wrapped, frozen tilapia fillets in the freezer and pull them out one at a time.

For adventurous eaters: easy lemon salmon with garlic spinach [17]

    4 salmon fillets—about 1 ½ pounds total (for 4 servings)

    4 teaspoons extra-virgin olive oil

    4 tablespoons lemon juice

    Salt and freshly ground pepper

    2 cloves garlic, chopped

    12 ounces baby spinach, rinsed

Line a baking sheet with foil and preheat broiler. If your oven doesn't contain a separate broiler, move rack to 5 to 6 inches below heating element.

Place fillets on the baking sheet and drizzle them evenly with 2 teaspoons olive oil and 2 tablespoons lemon juice. Sprinkle with salt and pepper to taste. Broil for 10 to 12 minutes or until cooked through.

Meanwhile, heat the remaining 2 teaspoons olive oil in a large skillet. Add the garlic and sauté, stirring, for 20 seconds. Add spinach, several handfuls at a time, and toss until each batch wilts and all 12 ounces fit into the skillet. Stir in the remaining 2 tablespoons lemon juice.

To serve, divide the spinach among 4 plates. Top each with a fillet.

Easy roasted vegetables

"Don't forget your vegetables!" How often have you heard your mother say those words? Well, she is right! Vegetables are low in fat, high in fiber and packed with nutrients!

Roasted tomatoes

To create a yummy veggie snack or side, try roasting a few tomatoes: the flavor is amazing! Cut plum or roma tomatoes in half and place them on a rimmed cookie sheet. Coat them with olive oil and sprinkle them with sea salt, freshly ground pepper and dried thyme. Roast at 425 degrees for about 20 minutes. If you desire, top them with a little feta cheese—a great addition!

Roasted broccoli

Toss broccoli florets in a bowl with 2 or 3 minced garlic cloves, 3 to 4 tablespoons olive oil, and 1 tablespoon lemon juice. Sprinkle with sea salt and freshly ground black pepper. Grease a baking sheet with olive oil and place the broccoli on the sheet. Bake at 425 degrees for 16 to 20 minutes until browned.

Roasted Brussels sprouts

Cut Brussels sprouts in half and place them on a baking sheet. Brush the sprouts with olive oil, and sprinkle them with sea salt and freshly ground pepper. Bake at 400 degrees for 25 to 30 minutes.

Nutrition tips

- Eat breakfast.
- Eat small meals throughout the day.
- Include a variety of lean protein.
- Include "good" carbohydrates: fruit, veggies and whole grains.
- Include Omega-3 fatty acids.
- Choose "good" unsaturated fats over "bad" saturated fats or trans fats.
- Drink lots of water.
- Limit white starchy carbohydrates.
- Go easy on the salt shaker.
- Avoid fried foods and cream sauces.
- Avoid processed foods.
- Limit sugary treats and drinks.
- Limit alcohol and caffeine.

Chips or fruit?

French fries or side salad?

Is this a good choice?

Am I really hungry?

? ?

?

CHAPTER 4
Emotional Eating
Versus
Mindful
Eating

**Change your brain and
reduce your flab!**

"FOOD is the most widely abused anti-anxiety drug in America, and EXERCISE is the most potent yet underutilized antidepressant."
—Bill Phillips

One of my clients, a young college student named Brittney, finally recognized that she was an emotional eater and did something about it. Here is her story:

> *Throughout my college career, I ate whenever I got emotionally upset and gained almost 60 pounds. I didn't know how to handle all my stress and got in the habit of overeating. At the time, I didn't realize I was gaining weight so rapidly. Somewhere along the line, I had lost the ability to feel full after eating a meal.*
>
> *Eventually the weight gain got to me enough that I took control of the situation by learning about nutrition and giving my body what it really needs. I trained myself to get out of the overeating habit. I learned what and how much of the different nutrients my body needs to help me feel full and feel fuller longer. Learning about nutrition has helped me live a healthier life. I have been losing weight and feel awesome.*
>
> *My overall goal is to live a healthy lifestyle and not think of this as a diet just to lose weight. It has been great to not treat my body like a trash can!*

Do you find yourself stuffing your face when you're not even hungry? Next time stop and think about what emotion you are feeling—exhaustion, boredom, anxiety, anger? If you try to find a solution for the emotion itself, you might save a lot of trips to kitchen and start shedding some pounds!

When I first used this technique, I was amazed at how often I was eating when I wasn't hungry. I remember going to the cupboard, stopping and asking myself, "Why am I here? I'm really not hungry!" I thought to myself, "What am I feeling?" I realized I was so tired that I wasn't motivated enough to do anything but walk around the kitchen and look for something to eat. My awareness allowed me to close the cupboard door, walk upstairs to my room, and lie down. Exhaustion was clearly a trigger to my emotional eating!

You can go as far as pinpointing very specific things in your life that cause you to rush to the refrigerator. Are you anxious because the guy you have been seeing hasn't called you in two days? Or is your math class a real struggle, causing frustration and worry? Maybe your parents are going through a divorce and you feel angry, hurt or helpless.

Regardless of the situation, many of us are emotional eaters, and it is extremely helpful to get in touch with our emotions and find the strength within ourselves to come up with solutions for specific issues in our life. Sometimes we can't solve the problem, but if that is the case, we must find better ways to deal with it. Why add to your negative emotions by making new ones with overeating?

Mindful eating techniques

Use mindful eating techniques and eat sloooowwwwly; don't forget to put on the brakes when you feel comfortably full. It takes 20 minutes for our bellies to tell us, "Hello! I feel good and satiated now!"

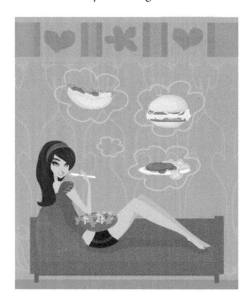

Think of your hunger on a scale from zero to ten, meaning that at one you are starving and at ten you are overly stuffed. Never let your hunger level get below a two. Eat a combination of protein, carbohydrates, and fat to bring you to about a seven on the hunger scale; hopefully you will stay satiated for about three to four hours and start over.

It's best to eat five or six small meals a day because you won't ever get to that "starving" feeling that can cause you to overeat and eat all the wrong things. I call this the Starve and Stuff Syndrome. It seems to make sense to save your appetite for that delicious dinner out or party where food will be served. However, going into a social gathering famished might very well cause you to eat the entire breadbasket at a restaurant or smorgasbord of finger foods at a party! Eat a little bit of lean protein before you go out and, you will eat fewer calories in the long run.

During one study, scientists fed two groups of people the same foods, which, of course, contained the same number of calories. The first group ate three meals a day. The second group ate small meals more often. The frequent eaters lost more weight. It is advantageous to keep your blood sugar stable throughout the day. Consequently, cravings will be reduced and the body will not go into a food storage mode, which plays havoc with the metabolism.

Do you take the time to really use your senses when you are eating? Try paying attention to the smell before you put it in your mouth. As you take a bite, notice the texture and analyze the taste. How many times have you chowed down at the computer and hardly remembered what you put in your mouth? That's no fun! Sit down, eat slowly and allow all of your senses to enjoy each bite without interruption. You are bound to eat less and feel more satisfied. Bon appetite!

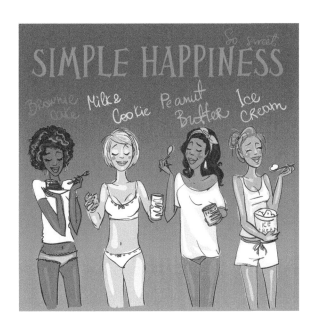

Binge buddies: friends who share the love of eating

Do you have binge buddies? You may not realize it, but if your roommate is eating a carton of ice cream on the couch, you may feel you have permission to do the same! How many times have you been with a group of friends whose entertainment was eating everything in sight or at least a lot of forbidden foods? It takes a lot of willpower to pick munchies like carrot sticks and apples when your friend pulls out the taco chips and cheese dip.

Recently my daughter sent me a picture of a salad she had made: chicken and veggies were beautifully arranged on a lovely plate. It looked like something you might be served at a great restaurant! I was shocked! I wondered if this was a joke. I had a hard time believing she had taken the time to create such an appealing, healthful meal.

The next day she sent me a text about a homemade soup she had made with chicken broth and veggies. As impressed as I was, I still could hardly believe it! What had gotten into my child, a college student? First of all, she is a junior, so she is out of the dorms and in an apartment with a kitchen. When I asked her more about her unusually healthy food choices, she said, "Karissa, my roommate taught me. She is really into healthy eating, and she's given me a ton of ideas!"

My daughter might not have been as motivated to prepare good food if she hadn't had a friend who was similarly motivated to eat well and stay in shape. When in high school, you may have heard your mother say, "You turn into your friends, so choose them wisely." You don't want to choose your friends based on their eating habits, but you can control the best environment in which to hang out with them. Always keep in the back of your mind that just because someone else is having a binge party, it doesn't make it OK for you! Your metabolism may not be as fast as your girlfriend's!

Don't turn eating into a sport or form of entertainment. For most of us, eating is far more fun than studying, but be careful with that! Ask yourself these questions:

- How are you feeling when you grab for forbidden foods?
- Are you paying attention to the size of your portions?
- Are you getting enough fruits, vegetables and lean protein?
- Are you drinking enough water?
- Are you taking in more calories than you thought?
- Do you realize how often you grab handfuls of empty calories?

Food logging

Logging one's food consumption for a few days can be very eye-opening: everyone should try it! If you use a smart phone app to log your foods, remember that a three-ounce portion of meat is about the size of a deck of cards or the palm of your hand, and a cup of pasta is about the size of a baseball or a fist. I recommend getting those little plastic portion cups or bowls from the grocery store that are labeled in cups or ounces so that you can determine amounts more accurately.

If you choose to log your food, you must include even the little things that sometimes add up to be the most calories. One client 'fessed up to me, "When I was logging all of my food, I was content with how many calories I recorded, but I wasn't losing any weight! What was I doing wrong? Oops, I never added the two packets of mayo I put on my sandwich, the tablespoon of butter I cooked my eggs in, and the creamer I put in my coffee. Now I have a clearer picture, and I'm watching the little things that really add up!"

Logging can be tedious, so do the best you can. It's impossible to be 100 percent accurate on portions sizes, and our memory sometimes fails us, but being diligent about it without expecting perfection, can go a long way! I tell some of my clients that if they prefer to record things later in the day, they can take a picture of their plate with their phone. Refer to serving equivalents in the nutrition chapter.

You might want to try using one of the following phone apps:[18]

- **Lose It!** (iPhone and Android: free) and **MyFitnessPal** (iphone, Android, BlackBerry and Windows: free) These apps have everything you need to track your food intake, especially if you are a data-driven person.

- **TrackNShare.** This app takes into account factors like mood or stress and how they affect eating behaviors. It is best for those who want a holistic or flexible approach to food journaling.

None of us want to obsess about our food intake, and my motto is, "Everything in moderation." In fact, give yourself permission to have a little naughty food occasionally. If 85 to 90 percent of your diet is wholesome, you are doing great. Deprivation and strict dieting causes bingeing in the long run. However, I will say that only a few days of paying closer attention with one of these apps will open your eyes to things you never realized!

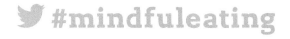

CHAPTER 5
Exercise

Control your stress, create a healthy high, and look better than ever.

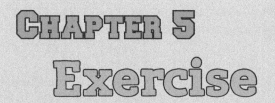

Change in activity may be the biggest factor causing college freshmen to gain weight, according to a study described in the *American Journal of Preventative Medicine*.[19] Current Physical Activity Guidelines recommend 150 minutes (or about 30 minutes, five times a week) of moderate to vigorous physical activity per week.

Many experts recommend longer durations of exercise—up to 60 minutes per day for weight loss.[20] To lose one pound, you have to decrease your caloric intake by 3,500 calories. For example, to lose two pounds a week, you have to increase caloric expenditure and decrease caloric intake by 500 calories a day. Many variables can affect this estimate, but regardless, the best way to lose weight is to burn more calories with added activity and reduce caloric intake by making better food choices. The combination of exercise and healthy eating habits gives you a much better chance of reaching your goals.

When you think of exercise, you may think of cardiovascular activity like running or using a step climber, treadmill or elliptical trainer. Aerobic exercise is an important component of exercise, especially to maintain a healthy weight and a healthy heart. However, resistance training is equally important! The goal is to change your body composition in addition to burning calories. With resistance training, we are able to do this. If you increase muscle, you will burn many more calories while just sitting there on Facebook and Instagram!

Muscles burn more calories than fat, even at rest. Weight-bearing exercise also helps build bone mass, which is imperative as we age. Some forms of cardiovascular exercise, like jogging, also have a weight-bearing advantage. Research shows that you can get a cardiovascular benefit from resistance training, as well.

Combining a well-rounded, strength-training program along with cardio training is the optimum way to go. You will also help prevent injury by strengthening the connective tissues and creating muscular balance. Turn your body into a fat-burning machine; goodbye muffin top, hello six-pack, and I'm talkin' abs not beer!

Exercise improves circulation and blood cholesterol levels. It also aids in preventing high blood pressure and bone loss. Physical activity is also one of the best treatments available for improved mental health. Both resistance and cardiovascular activity are proven to alleviate symptoms of anxiety and depression, as well as contributing to higher levels of self-esteem and energy. Exercise increases the flow of oxygen, which directly affects the brain and promotes mental sharpness and improved memory.[21] What college student couldn't use a little dose of mental sharpness topped with a memory enhancer, drug free?

When you are young, often the main motivation to exercise is to improve your physical appearance, which I do admit is an added bonus! But please recognize and remember that every minute of physical activity you engage in now will not only contribute to your best bikini body but will also help lead you to good health, happiness and success.

Without healthy eating and exercise, your mental and physical health could steadily decline and the odds that disease and injury will come knocking at your door are greatly increased! Don't take the "all or nothing" approach, either. It is amazing how many ways you can squeeze exercise into spare minutes throughout the day.

When the coffee is brewing, do a set of 10 to 15 pushups against the counter. When you are waiting for your roommate to get out of the shower, try another set or advance to the carpet and do a set of pushups from your knees. Pop off a few after you get out of the shower. It's amazing how you can tone your arms, chest, shoulders and upper back and even gain core strength with a simple pushup! You can similarly tone your legs by doing squats while you brush your teeth or take a study break.

And girl, why would you drive to class if it's less than a mile or two away? If you only walk half a mile to and from class, four days a week, you will rack up four miles a week, sixteen miles a month! If there is a gym on campus, why not read your homework assignment while you are on the stationary bike?

Create micro workouts combining aerobic and resistance training while you watch television. The key to getting started is knowing the exercises and the muscles working, in addition to proper form and balanced routines.

Resistance workouts for your dorm room

Below are descriptions and photos of some balanced, strength-training workouts that will tone your entire body. You can do these exercises in a dorm room, bedroom or small apartment. All you need is your body weight and a pair of supportive workout shoes. Even clothes are optional!

If you want a variation, invest in a pair or two of dumbbells. Keep your weight-lifting motion slow and controlled. You want that last rep to challenge you, so work it, baby! Remember this principle: if you're using momentum to complete the exercise, the weight is too heavy. An example of this would be if you are throwing your torso backward while you are doing a bicep curl.

Finally, make sure you get a doctor's clearance if you have any medical issues or physical injuries.

Important tip: Take the time to learn the major muscles and the exercises that strengthen them. I have added descriptions to each photo to help you with that. Think about the muscles you are working, and the correct exercise position will fall into place.

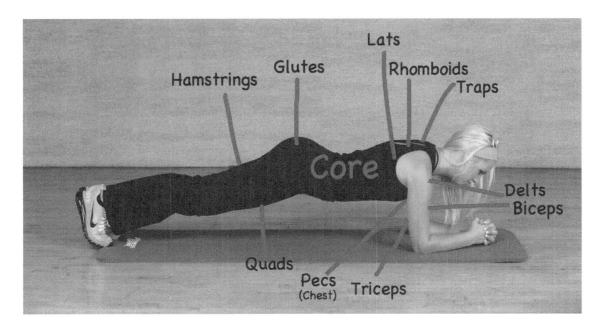

Deltoids: muscles that form your shoulder.

Biceps: muscles in the front of your upper arm.

Triceps: muscles in the back of your upper arm.

Pectoralis muscles (pecs): muscles in the chest area.

Latissimus Dorsi (lats): fan-shaped muscles on the lateral sides of the mid-back area.

Rhomboids: muscles in the middle, upper back.

Trapezius: a triangular muscle in the upper back, shoulder and neck area.

Gluteals: muscles that make up your butt.

Hamstrings: muscles in the back of your upper leg.

Quadriceps(quads): muscles in the front of your upper leg.

The importance of core work

Your "core" is the midsection of your body. The condition of your core muscles affects the entire body function like a chain reaction. A strong core will aid and support the other areas of your body, reducing injury. Abdominal and low back exercises, including planks, are essential to your strength training program. When spring break comes, you will be thanking me for that six pack!

The importance of warming up

Warming up is imperative! Getting that blood flowing to the muscles will increase the quality of your workout and prevent injury. I know many people learn that the hard way. Twenty-somethings are not imune to injury! Just last week my twenty-year-old son was taken by amulance to the hospital due to back muscle spasms that hit him during his workout. We all have weak areas and imbalances in our bodies. The older you get, the more you will recognize them. Three to five minutes of jumping jacks, jogging in place, or dancing is a must before your workout.

The importance of stretching

Most people do not take the time to stretch as they should. It's not until they pull a muscle, or feel tight in some spots, that they actually realize the importance of stretching. Aside from preventing injury, your range of motion will increase, aiding your workout and athletic abilities. The most important time to stretch is after your workout. However, doing some simple stretches after your warm up and before your workout can be helpful. Never stretch a cold muscle! Please don't ignore the stretching section of this chapter. I kept it simple, so go for it!

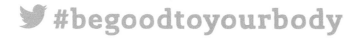 #begoodtoyourbody

Ten-minute body-weight strength workout

- Warm up 3 to 5 minutes
  1. **Pushup from knees**
     Targets chest and works front shoulder, arms and core.
     Start with arms straight and hands shoulder width apart. Lower nose and chest to floor. Repeat 10 to 15 times.

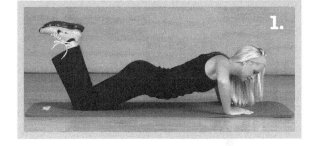

  2. **Squat**
     Targets hamstrings, glutes and quadriceps.
     Start in standing position. Lower legs as if sitting on a chair and push up through the heels. Don't allow knees to extend passed toes. Repeat 10 to 20 times. For extra credit: add 10 tiny presses in the lower position!

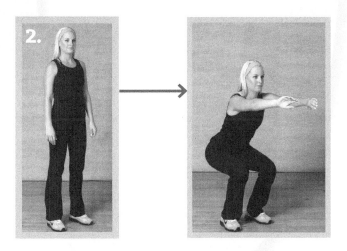

3. **Abdominal curl up**
Targets your abdominal muscles.
Lie on your back with elbows out and hands at ears. Contract abdominals by raising shoulders off the floor without pulling on the neck. Repeat 10 to 15 times.

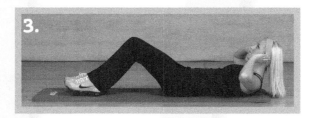

4. **Low back extension**
Targets the low back, but also hits the glutes!

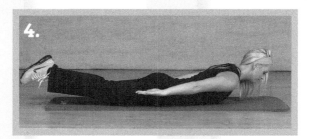

In prone position (face down), raise chest off the floor and hold 5 seconds, lower and repeat up to 10 times.

- Repeat sequence two to three times.
- Stretch.

Fifteen-minute body-weight workout

1. **Lunge**

   Targets the quadriceps, hamstrings and gluteals.
   Start in a standing position and lower body. Try not to let the knee extend over toe. Push up through the heel and repeat 10 to 20 times. Repeat on the other side. For extra credit: add 10 tiny presses in the lower position!

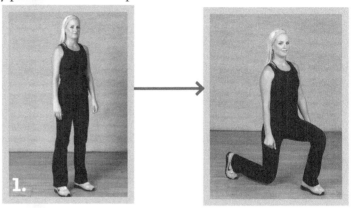

2. **Plank**

   Targets the core, but works the entire body!
   Rotate your hips left and right or lift and pulse one leg up and down for an advanced plank alternative. Hold body in a straight plain for 30 to 60 seconds.

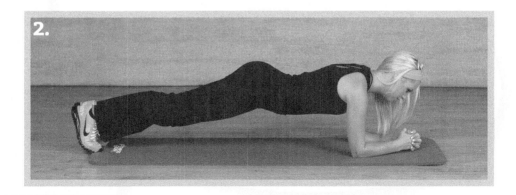

3. **Rotating side plank**
Targets the core, but works the whole body!
Start in side plank and rotate onto the other hand, hold for two seconds and repeat for a total of 15 to 20 rotations. Lift leg up and down between rotations for an advanced movement.

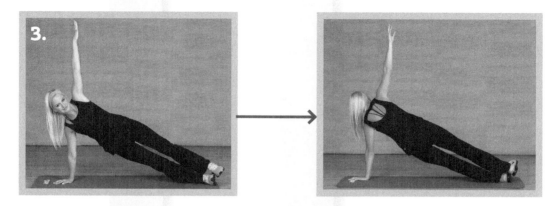

4. **Tricep dip**
Targets the triceps.
Lower your body by bending at the elbow. Push up using your triceps and repeat 10 to 15 times. For a more advanced version, straighten your legs.

- Repeat sequence 2 to 3 times.
- Stretch.

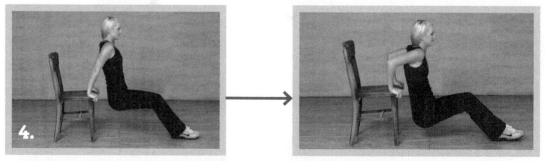

20-minute body-weight workout

1. **Pushup**
   Targets the pecs (chest) and works additional muscles such as upper back and triceps.
   Start with arms straight, lower down and press up through your upper body. Repeat 10 to 15 times.

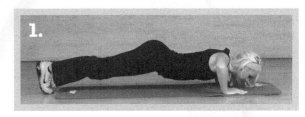

2. **Boat pose**
   Targets the core muscles.
   Hold for 30 to 60 seconds.

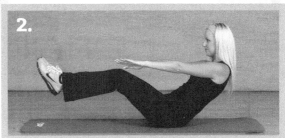

3. **Bicycle abdominal crunch**
   Targets the abdominal muscles.
   Twist upper body, pointing elbow to opposite knee. Alternate without pulling on your neck. Repeat 20 times.

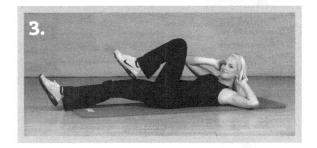

4. **Hip abduction**
   Targets outer thigh muscles.
   Raise top leg up and down. Keep toe facing forward. Use an ankle weight or band for more resistance. Repeat 10 to 20 times per side.

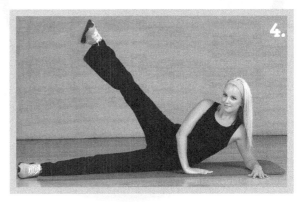

5. Hip adduction
Targets the inner thigh muscles.
Raise lower leg up and down. Repeat 10 to 20 times per side.

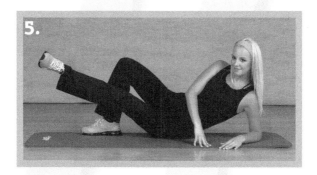

6. Hell raiser
Targets the quadriceps.
Put feet flat against the wall. Start with knees bent. Extend legs, then Lower. Repeat 10 to 20 times.

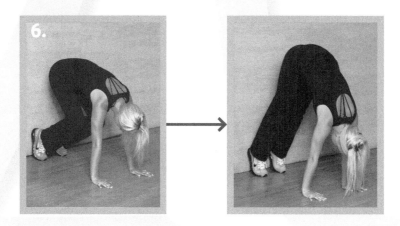

7. **Glute bridge**

Targets the gluteal and hamstring muscles.
Lie on your back with knees bent. Raise hips up, hold for two seconds,
then lower. Repeat 10 to 20 times.

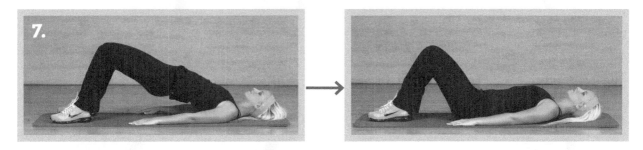

8. **Bird dog**

Targets the low back muscles and engages the glutes and abdominals.
Start on hands and knees. Extend arm and opposite leg, hold for a few seconds,
and repeat.

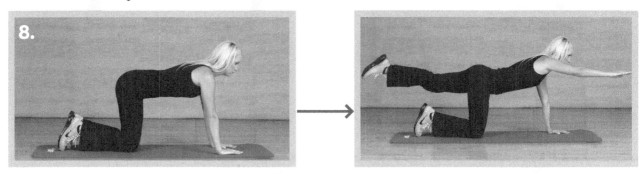

- Repeat sequence two to three times.
- Stretch.

Upper-body exercises with weights

(I recommend purchasing a set of 5 and 10 pound weights to start.)

- Perform 2 to 3 sets of 10 to 15 reps.

1. **Chest press**
   Targets the pecs (chest).
   Hold arms at a 90-degree angle and extend arms up to meet at the top, then lower. Repeat 10 to 15 times.

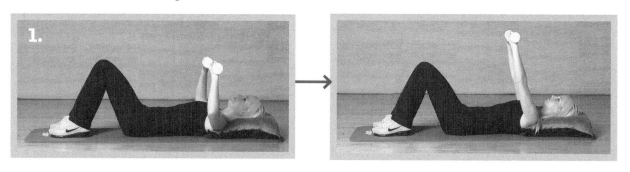

2. **Bentover back row**
   Targets the lats.
   Lean over with a flat back. Pull elbows back,
   squeeze shoulder blades together, then lower. Repeat 10 to 15 times.

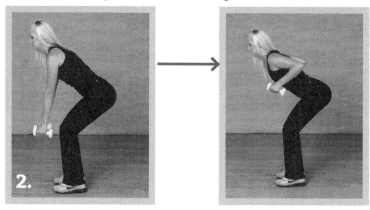

3. Shoulder press

Targets the delts (shoulders).

Stand with arms at a ninety-degree angle and extend arms overhead, then lower. Repeat 10 to 15 times.

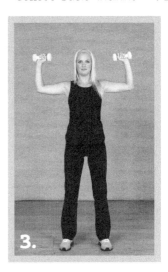

4. Bicep curl

Targets the biceps.

Start with weights at your side and curl up, then lower. Repeat 10 to 15 times.

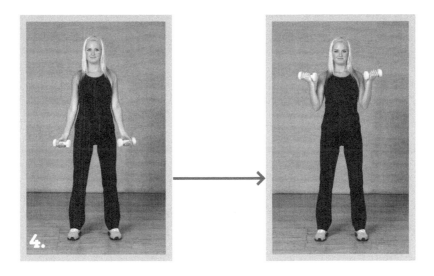

5. Tricep kickback
Targets the triceps.
Raise elbow to high position and hold while kicking back the weight. Hinge at the elbow while holding the upper arms still. Repeat 10 to 15 times.

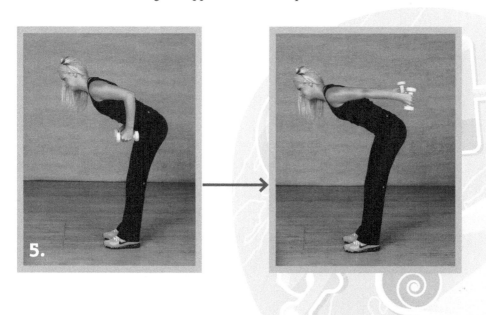

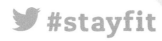

Lower body exercises with weights

1. **Lunge with weights**
   Repeat 10 to 15 times.

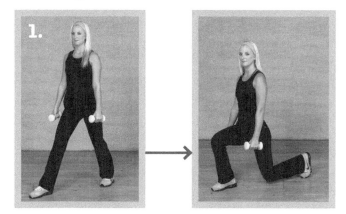

2. **Squat with weights**
   Repeat 10 to 15 times.

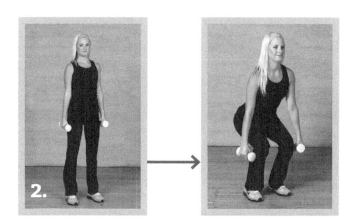

3. **Glute bridge with weights**
   Repeat 10 to 15 times.

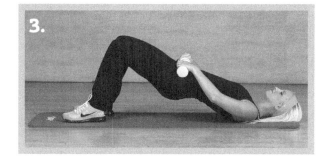

Stretches

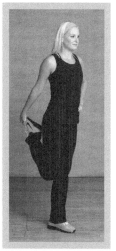

Quadricep stretch

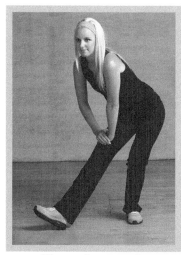

Hamstring stretch

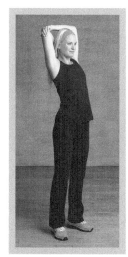

Tricep stretch

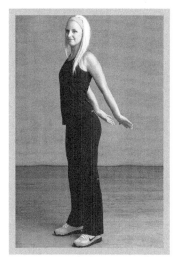

Bicep and chest stretch

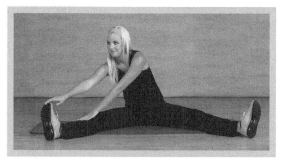

Inner-thigh stretch

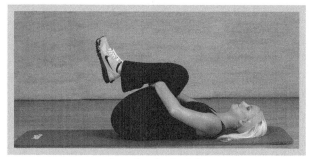

Low-back stretch

Food and fluids for fitness

It's important to drink water before, during and after your workout to stay hydrated. Starting your workout in a dehydrated state will not allow you to work out at your best, and replenishing throughout and afterwards is important because you will lose water as you perspire.

Before the workout

Don't count on last night's dinner to fuel you for a morning workout. If you plan on exercising within an hour of eating, choose a light snack rather than a full breakfast. It's important to put the emphasis on carbohydrates for energy, but it might be advantageous to have a little protein, as well. Light meals or snacks might include a banana or whole-grain toast with peanut butter, yogurt, milk with whole-grain cereal, or protein shakes with fruit.

The general rule is to eat large meals three to four hours before exercising, small meals two to three hours before, and small snacks an hour before exercising. It's tough to work out when you haven't consumed some energy because you will have no energy to expend; the result is feeling weak and sometimes shaky. On the other hand, if you eat too much, you might feel sluggish or even develop stomach issues.

After the workout

After a workout we want to refuel so that we help our muscles recover and replace glycogen stores. Experts recommend eating a meal that contains both protein and carbohydrates within a couple of hours of exercise. Sandwiches with meat, string cheese and apples, nuts and dried fruit, or a regular meal that includes a meat, starch and cooked vegetable or salad are examples of effective choices.

How much

How much you should eat before and after exercise depends on whether you are training for marathons or walking a couple of miles. The intensity of your exercise will dictate how much and how often you eat. Make sure to get a combination of protein and carbohydrates at each meal, and eat until you are comfortably full; don't let your hunger get so intense that you are ravenous.

If you are participating in a resistance-training program, you might want to increase your protein intake to help build and repair muscle. Finally, don't forget to stay hydrated with plenty of water. For those who train intensely for more than 60 minutes, sports drinks can help maintain the body's electrolyte balance.

Each of us is an individual, so pay attention to how you feel and what works for you. Try logging the foods and time that you eat before you exercise. After your workout, log how you felt during the workout. Soon you will identify what works for you!

CHAPTER 6
Eating Disorders

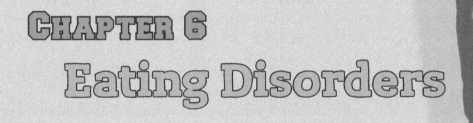

Are you—or is someone you know—in danger because of fighting with food?

Eating disorders are conditions in which individuals have an intense, detrimental preoccupation with food and weight. A young woman named Krista, like many others, had a severe battle with food but courageously managed to overcome it. Here is her story:

> I was the girl who had everything but felt nothing. I was a young, blooming blonde who fulfilled many high school dreams and aspirations and excelled in a variety of activities. However, managing academic requirements, creating a social life, and participating in a varsity athletic team and other organizations became a challenge. Teachers, administrators, counselors and coaches pushed and pulled me in different directions. Each focused on his or her expertise, of course. I became overwhelmed.

> I have always had strong morals and values. However, the "popular" group that I became a part of represented the complete opposite of my beliefs. I liked belonging to this group, which seemed glamorous. I enjoyed the attention and had fun, but looking back I see I was definitely in the wrong place. Deep down, I didn't really know who I was.

> Relationships became heartbreaking in high school. Because I was the "good girl," I was kicked to the curb. It was hard to understand.

> When I got to college, I wanted to find new friends and take on a new life. However, I found I had a closed mind. Growing up in the suburbs, I had become accustomed to one type of lifestyle and had not been exposed to diversity. As I slowly adapted to the environment and became open to people of different backgrounds, I met a boy who taught me not to judge others so quickly. He was a small-town guy who enjoyed the little things in life. He loved me and made me happy, but I had questions. He was not the man I pictured in my future.

> I soon became insecure and constantly compared myself to other girls in this boy's life. I also questioned the direction of my academics. All this turmoil came on quickly. I started to criticize myself and tried to become the "perfect girl" that everyone thought I was—the girl who had everything and looked glamorous. I put a lot of pressure on myself.

> My boyfriend began changing. I felt as if his eyes were looking past me. I became depressed, tense and irritable. I blamed him for my depression and

irritability. I broke up with him and tried to start a new life. I had no idea who I was or where I was heading.

I looked at pictures on Facebook and became angry with myself because of the way I looked. I was a little bigger and hated it. I wanted to do something about it. So many emotions built up that I just exploded and headed on a mission to lose weight. I thought that if I became more confident about my body, I would be happier.

I worked out every day and ate a very restricted diet. The idea of a perfect body got into my head and nearly destroyed me. I was lost and felt sick every time I thought about my former boyfriend. I missed the comfort of having someone. My eating and pursuit of fitness spiraled out of control. When I looked into the mirror, I no longer saw reality. All I saw was a lonely, overweight female.

I started to make myself sick when I ate something I thought I shouldn't eat. My body shook because it craved certain foods I wouldn't allow myself to eat. Once in a while I broke my own rules and instantly became so upset with myself I would throw up.

I became crabby and snappy and got annoyed easily. I started to have anxiety attacks. I would get myself so worked up that my entire body would shake and I would hyperventilate. Once I even passed out. One night my anger at myself became so intense I didn't want to live anymore. It was all too much to handle. My head was bursting and my body shaking. I realized the situation was dangerous and went to the hospital psych ward.

I finally asked for help. It was the hardest thing I have ever done. I met with two psychiatrists, but they could not help me because I cherry-coated my status and was not open-minded during the sessions. I did not want to take medicine. I wanted to do everything on my own.

Doctors prescribed five medications for anxiety and depression. Some of them caused severe reactions, and I had to discontinue them. I tried counseling, but it didn't work. During this time I was just drained, emotionally and physically. I was also extremely selfish and wanted to do things my way. My weight dropped to 100 pounds. I was not fun to be around.

Eventually, I had to go to a doctor for a checkup, and that is when I finally came to terms with everything. He explained to me that it is OK to get help and take medications. He said, "You are not any weaker than anyone else because you take medications. No one is perfect." I realized I had been striving to become that "perfect" person who had everything.

I started to take my medication regularly. However, I knew taking pills was not going to solve everything. I had to do my homework. I returned to my doctors and was able to talk through my disease. I took on hobbies and kept myself focused on what really mattered—the loved ones around me.

Every day I took a small step to a better me. I put all my energy into what I felt deep down inside. I listened to my heart instead of the outside world. I now have overcome the disease and proved to everyone that the real me was there.

I found my truth through mentors and loved ones and by taking my medication religiously. I now live a new life I am proud of. I surround myself with people who lift my spirits. I am blessed to have found amazing girlfriends in college. Each and every one of them has had a huge influence on my life. I finally realized I am not alone in this world.

—Krista, age 21

The moral of this story is clear: if you have an eating disorder, don't try to solve all your problems yourself. Get professional help, the sooner the better. Your life is infinitely valuable, not only to yourself but to all the people who love you.

Trying to lose weight?

If you are trying to lose weight, do it the healthy way: don't lose more than two pounds a week, and achieve this goal by moderately reducing calorie intake and increasing daily activity and exercise. Losing weight takes time. As I mentioned earlier, it takes a reduction of 3,500 calories to lose a single pound. Many of us are not patient enough and resort to extreme measures to lose weight quickly. Eventually some of these behaviors blow up into full-fledged eating disorders. You may not realize how dangerous that is.

How many of you have decided you need a quick fix? It's Wednesday and you need to get into the skintight dress by Saturday night. "I'll just fast for a few days," you tell yourself. However, when you abruptly withdraw all nutrients from your body, detrimental things occur. Will a few days create a serious problem? Maybe not, but over time the body will make modifications to compensate for the lost nutrition.

You may lose weight initially, but your body will go into survival mode, causing a drop in your basal metabolic rate, which means you will need fewer calories to survive. Consequently, you

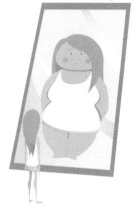

will also lose lean body mass and create nutritional deficiencies. The last thing you want to do is slow down your metabolism! Instead, increase your activity and moderately lower your caloric intake with healthier choices and portion control.

Eating disorders are very serious. Most young people think it's no big deal to stop eating, because if you start to feel weak and sick, you can just put fuel back into your body, and it will be OK! This is not always the case. Sometimes the damage that has been done by starving oneself is irreversible and death ensues. This is serious stuff! No "skinny" goal is worth a life.

We are all built differently. We have to embrace our natural shapes, respect our bodies, and be assured that perfection does not exist. Sometimes life throws us a curve ball, and our minds trick us into thinking that our self-worth is all wrapped up in our appearance. When these negative thoughts overwhelm us and cause us to do things we know are not healthy, it's time to seek medical help.

School health services and medical doctors deal with eating disorders every day. These disorders are nothing to be ashamed of. They are simply a common problem that most often needs some kind of medical treatment. Your primary doctor will be able to refer you to a reputable qualified practitioner or counselor who will lead you in the right direction.

The three main types of eating disorders are anorexia nervosa, bulimia nervosa and binge-eating disorder. Here are the definitions, symptoms and red flags associated with each of these disorders, as identified by the Mayo Clinic:[22]

Anorexia nervosa

When you have anorexia nervosa, you're obsessed with food and being thin, sometimes to the point of deadly self-starvation. Symptoms of anorexia nervosa are:

- Refusal to eat and denial of hunger
- An intense fear of gaining weight
- A negative or distorted self-image
- Excessive exercise
- Flat mood or lack of emotion
- Irritability
- Fear of eating in public

- Preoccupation with food
- Social withdrawal
- Thin appearance
- Trouble sleeping
- Soft, downy hair present on the body (lanugo)
- Menstrual irregularities or loss of menstruation (amenorrhea)
- Constipation
- Abdominal pain
- Dry skin
- Frequently being cold
- Irregular heart rhythms
- Low blood pressure
- Dehydration

Bulimia nervosa

When you have bulimia, you have episodes of bingeing and purging. During these episodes, you typically eat a large amount of food in a short duration and then try to rid yourself of the extra calories through vomiting or excessive exercise. You may be at a normal weight or even a bit overweight. Symptoms of bulimia may include:

- Eating until the point of discomfort or pain, often with high-fat or sweet foods
- Self-induced vomiting
- Laxative use
- Excessive exercise
- An unhealthy focus on body shape and weight
- A distorted, excessively negative body image
- Low self-esteem
- Going to the bathroom after eating or during meals
- A feeling that you can't control your eating behavior
- Abnormal bowel functioning
- Damaged teeth and gums
- Swollen salivary glands in the cheeks
- Sores in the throat and mouth
- Dehydration
- Irregular heartbeat
- Sores, scars or calluses on the knuckles or hands
- Menstrual irregularities or loss of menstruation (amenorrhea)

- Constant dieting or fasting
- Possibly, drug and alcohol abuse

Binge-eating disorder

When you have binge-eating disorder, you regularly eat excessive amounts of food (binge), but don't try to compensate for this behavior with exercise or purging as someone with bulimia or anorexia might. You may eat when you're not hungry and continue eating even long after you are uncomfortably full. After a binge, you may feel guilty or ashamed, which can trigger a new round of bingeing. You may be a normal weight, overweight or obese. Symptoms of binge-eating disorder may include:

- Eating to the point of discomfort or pain
- Eating much more food during a binge episode than during a normal meal or snack
- Eating faster during binge episodes
- Feeling that your eating behavior is out of control
- Frequently eating alone
- Feeling depressed, disgusted or upset over the amount eaten

Because of its powerful pull, an eating disorder can be difficult to manage or overcome by yourself. Eating disorders can virtually take over your life. You may think about food all the time, spend hours agonizing over what to eat, and exercise to exhaustion. You may feel ashamed, sad, hopeless, drained, irritable and anxious. You may also have a host of physical problems such as irregular heartbeats, fatigue, and bowel or menstrual troubles.[23]

Red flags that may indicate an eating disorder include:

- Skipping meals
- Making excuses for not eating
- Eating only a few certain "safe" foods, usually those low in fat and calories
- Adopting rigid meal or eating rituals, such as cutting food into tiny pieces or spitting food out after chewing
- Cooking elaborate meals for others, but refusing to eat them themselves
- Collecting recipes
- Withdrawing from normal social activities
- Persistent worry or complaining about being fat
- A distorted body image, such as complaining about being fat despite being underweight

- Not wanting to eat in public
- Frequent checking in the mirror for perceived flaws
- Wearing baggy or layered clothing
- Repeatedly eating large amounts of sweet or high-fat foods
- Use of syrup of ipecac, laxatives, the over-the-counter weight-loss drug Orlistat (Alli), or over-the-counter drugs that can cause fluid loss, such as menstrual symptom relief medications
- Use of dietary supplements or herbal products for weight loss
- Hoarding food
- Leaving during meals to use the toilet
- Eating in secret

It's important to realize what a normal weight is and not go to the media for comparisons to unrealistic models. Try not to engage in social media or websites that promote disordered eating. It's easy to fall back into dangerous habits or justify those habits if you are exposing yourself to sites and people who glorify it. It is amazing what professional Photoshop users can do to perfect any human being! Those women and men are far from perfect, just like you and me. They can lengthen legs, flatten tummies and perfect skin so they are baby flawless!

Positive role models are very important at this stage. Choose them carefully! Be aware of triggers, and have a plan in place so that you can deal with them positively. Keeping a journal that includes your emotions and behaviors can be very beneficial in developing self-awareness. Finally, realize that recovery takes time. It's very important to stick with the support you are receiving for the recommended time.[24]

For more information and support regarding eating disorders,
go to http://www.NationalEatingDisorders.org/

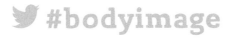 #bodyimage

CHAPTER 7
Depression and Anxiety

Do you—or does someone you know—feel out of control emotionally?

We can't always control what happens to us and how we handle things. However, most of us, with the proper help, are able to work through even life's toughest challenges. This college girl admitted to me she was experiencing anxiety stemming from a traumatic experience four years earlier:

> When I was 16, I was involved in a drinking and driving accident. I didn't know how to deal with this awful event or handle my emotions. I just tried to push the whole upsetting episode out of my mind. Later in my life, these emotions surfaced. I started to suffer from panic attacks, which I tried to control with caffeine and alcohol. Both of these substances had very negative impacts: they just increased the level of my anxiety.
>
> Eventually I got the medical help I needed, and I have learned to live and deal with anxiety in a constructive way. Medication, proper nutrition, yoga and exercise have had a positive impact on my whole outlook on life.

Depression and anxiety

Are you wondering if you or a friend is suffering from depression or anxiety? These very common mood disorders can affect all aspects of one's daily life. Clinical depression is characterized by at least two weeks of depressed mood or loss of interest in most activities that the person formerly enjoyed.[25]

Generalized anxiety disorder (GAD) is characterized by excessive anxiety and worry about a number of events or situations on most days, for at least six months.[26] Often people have a combination of both anxiety and depression.

Suzanne, a client of mine, recently told me a story about her son that illustrates the anguish of such a situation:

> When my son was a senior in high school, he became depressed and lost all motivation to work hard in school. He simply didn't care. His sports had always been the most important thing in his life, but during this time he just quit his lacrosse team. Nothing mattered to him. It was if a switch had been flipped and nothing made him happy. He felt sad and hopeless and was often irritable. The consequences of failing his classes or getting into legal trouble were of no threat to him because he didn't value his life: in his mind, risk-taking was not even a risk.
>
> Was I afraid he was going to hurt himself? Absolutely! Would anyone else

who knew him believe this could be happening to a responsible, popular, all-American boy who "had it all"? Absolutely not! What caused this change? I don't know. I'm not sure even he knows what started this downward spiral.

However, I do know there were stressors in his life. School was challenging, sports weren't going as well as he had hoped, and the anticipation and fear of transitioning from high school to college was brewing, whether he knew it consciously or not.

We have all heard the term "hitting rock bottom." When a vulnerable person is experiencing a bout of depression, days, hours and even minutes can be filled with risk. One moment of desperation can lead to a life-threatening situation. Thank goodness we were able to get help for our son before some tragedy occurred.

Depression and anxiety can range from mild to severe, but regardless, it's not something we want to ignore. Many of us have been touched by a family member, friend or friend of a friend who has attempted or committed suicide. It's a very real problem in society today, but it can be avoided if depression is caught and treated before it's too late.

College students are experiencing more difficult transitions than ever before. They must adjust to new places to live, new friends, changes in identity, budget concerns, and higher levels of responsibilities and academic stress.

 There is no shame in admitting to others that life isn't perfect. Talking about your feelings might make others feel that they are not the only ones who are struggling! Catch your discomfort while you can function rationally, or help a friend before the risks become threatening.

Don't hesitate to call a trusted adult. People who are struggling with depression or anxiety often are calling for help in their own way. Young adults sometimes have this idea that you must never call "the adults" because you don't want to "throw your friend under the bus!" Guess what, my friend? This isn't junior high anymore. Now YOU are the adult! The risks can be incomprehensible. Get help for yourself or a friend in need. Call a mother, brother, sister, teacher, father, aunt or uncle—anyone with whom you feel comfortable.

Often anxiety and depression are all rolled up into one! Symptoms of both are listed below. However, rather than getting caught up in an exact diagnosis, try to recognize the signs indicating when help is necessary. That is what's important. You are smart and have a good gut feeling. If things are not right, do what you can to help yourself or someone else.

Symptoms of depression or anxiety may include:[27]

- Changes in appetite
- Sleep disturbances
- Low energy
- Agitation
- Trouble concentrating
- Difficulty in making decisions
- Feelings of hopelessness and sadness
- Feeling worthless or guilty
- Easily tearing up or crying when talking about emotions
- Excessive worry
- Feelings of restlessness
- Easily fatigued
- Irritability
- Muscle tension

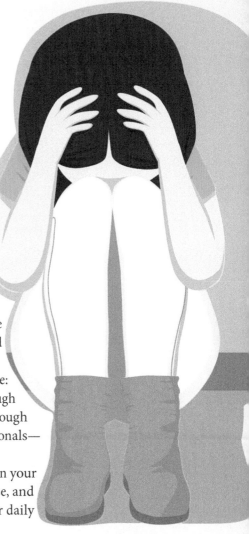

Students sometimes hesitate to make a connection with the mental health office of the college they attend. Lots of people need mental health advice at one time or another.

Walking into any counseling office is not the walk of shame: it's the walk of success. Just as academic counselors guide you through your curriculum, health service employees can guide you through physical illness, and mental health counselors—trained professionals— can help you get through the temporary stresses of college life.

Over time, stress can have a tremendously negative impact on your body. Make sure you get plenty of sleep, good nutrition and exercise, and keep in mind the following ideas that may help you cope with your daily life:

- Get emotional support from a trusted friend, family member or counselor. Don't be afraid to get answers to your questions, whether they pertain to academic or emotional issues. Be proactive about maintaining a support system.

- Make time for the passions or interests that bring you joy and relaxation, even if that duration of time is just a couple of hours a week.

- Don't overload yourself. Try to be conscious of what you as an individual can handle, depending on your own situation. If you make a scheduling mistake, recognize that it is not shameful to drop a class: it happens!

- Try some forms of deep breathing or meditation simply by sitting in a quiet room and inhaling deeply through your nose and exhaling slowly through your mouth. There are many smart phone apps that assist with breathing and relaxation. Download a podcast app and search the options! Plug in your headphones and escape into a world of relaxation for a brief time. This technique also helps if you have trouble sleeping. Sometimes when tensions build and muscles get tight, a professional massage therapist can help you decompress![28]

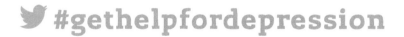 **#gethelpfordepression**

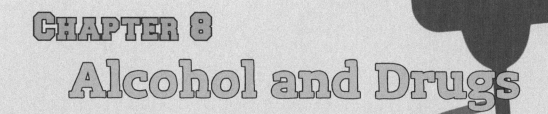

CHAPTER 8
Alcohol and Drugs

"YOLO!" Let the "pregaming"
begin . . . or not. Proceed
with caution!

When you drink, do you feel relaxed? Are you the life of the party? Do you feel all your stress go away? Do you feel invincible? Oh, yeah, drinking can be a lot of fun, aid you in some social interaction you might not otherwise partake in, and create some great stories! But beware . . .

Here is a true story about how one young woman made a bad decision about how much to drink and found herself in the midst of a nightmare:

> It was a typical Friday night, and one of my college friends was throwing a party. I had a bad cold and should have stayed in, but I really wanted to go because I knew my boyfriend would be there, and I wanted to see him.

> I didn't feel as if I drank very much, but I ended up extremely drunk, likely due to mixing alcohol with cold medicine. We were all having a great time. However, as I drove home alone afterward, it was raining really hard, and I could barely see. I missed a turn and ran into something. My airbags went off, and my first instinct was to get out and run. I remember tripping and falling and being so scared!

> I soon heard sirens and thought to myself, "What have I done?" The police showed up and gave me a sobriety test. They then sat me in the cop car and made me take a Breathalyzer. A million thoughts ran through my head, but I told myself not to cry. That is when they told me I was under arrest for a DWI.

> A police officer drove me past the scene where my car was, but all I could see were people and flashing lights. The officer took me to the police station, where I was questioned and fingerprinted.

> I called my mom. When I saw her for the first time, I was sobbing uncontrollably because I could see in her face how disappointed she was. That was when someone told me I had run my car into someone's house. Mom couldn't even talk to me the whole time she was driving home.

> When I woke up the next morning, I was in much pain from the impact of the airbags. And I had no feelings of emotion at all. I was completely numb and in shock. My family was so sad. It felt like someone in our family had died.

> My dad drove me to the house where the accident happened. It was shocking to see the damage I had caused. The homeowner kept saying she was glad I

was OK. Then she added, "The damage can be fixed but losing someone is irreversible." I apologized for everything I had done. She said her wish for me was that I learn from this experience. I was overwhelmed with guilt and shame. It was hard to talk to anyone.

After going back to college, I found out how fast word travels. I was identified as the drunk who ran into the house. When my court date came along, I wanted to represent myself and plead guilty. The judge looked at me and said he was giving me two years of unsupervised probation with the charge of a misdemeanor DWI. He said he was letting me off easy and he didn't want to see my face in that courtroom again because I wouldn't be given a second chance. I also had to do community service, and I lost my license for 18 months.

Many people lost respect for me and were disappointed in my choices. I told myself I had to pay this all off and take it as a learning experience. Today I am grateful I have learned from my mistakes and have become a more driven, hardworking, independent person. I think God wanted more for me than the dark path down which I was headed.

—Brittney, age 19

Dangers of binge drinking and recreational drugs

Aside from the fact that getting "wasted" is really hard on your body, it causes a lot of trouble! One college student was reflecting on his drinking experience:

Everything seems like a really good idea when you have been drinking too much. When I have my beer goggles on, all women are sexy. One night after drinking too much, I took a girl home, and I thought she was a ten. When I woke up, she was definitely a two. AWKWARD!

Creative ideas flourish, confidence rises, judgment flies out the window, most members of the opposite sex look hot, fear of danger is nonexistent, losing your phone or wallet is a standard, and overeating is the norm. I would like to know the true statistics of how many students have lost their phones during their freshman year, most often to snow banks and toilets.

A friend of mine was shocked to find out that her son David was a victim of theft perpetrated by his own longtime, childhood friend. While David and his fraternity brothers were all partying it up, the friend stole David's cash card from his room and had a heyday at Target! Theft is prevalent in college, trust me, and it's a lot easier to commit this crime when everyone is drunk or high and not paying attention.

A student I knew had a lot to drink and, rather than joining her group at a bar and drinking more, she chose to crash at her friend's apartment. Good decision, right? A male roommate of the friend came home and took advantage of the situation by sexually assaulting her. Her memory was fuzzy, and justice was very hard to achieve.

Another student I knew—a bright young man from a responsible family—had a tendency to fight when he drank too much. He picked a fight with another kid and smashed a bottle over his head. Charges were pressed, the story was all over the news, and the aggressor was kicked out of college with an assault record. While under the influence of alcohol, even "nice kids" can turn into violent drunks. Futures can be destroyed, and families can be crushed.

A college athlete I met got into a drinking altercation and gently pushed a guy on a bike, so he thought! The man on the bike, who was also intoxicated, loss control and hit a brick wall. He lay in a coma for days until he finally died. Suddenly a young college student was dead and a very decent college athlete who had no prior record was facing murder charges. Needless to say, he was also kicked out of college and off the school's sports teams.

Mixing alcohol and the bitter cold winter nights can be dangerous. One female student was dropped off at the wrong house late one night after an evening of partying. When she was looking for her house she got confused and passed out on a stranger's porch. The resident found her the next morning almost frozen to death. As I write these words, she remains in critical condition and will likely lose her limbs.

A week later a young college freshman was found frozen to death along the riverbank near a University of Minnesota campus. No one knows for sure what happened to him, but his buddies were with him at a party, last seeing him at 12:30 a.m. It appears as though he left a party alone, fell on his way home, hit his head, and tumbled down a steep hill in subzero weather. The grief this family and his young friends are going through is incomprehensible for most. One wrong turn, one too many drinks, one bad decision and the life of a beautiful young man with a bright future, a loving family and hundreds of friends, is over.

There are numerous stories about students getting hit and killed by vehicles along roads and at crosswalks at night. Some of the drivers are the distracted ones, but often the walkers are under the influence and not looking before they cross the street. We always think of little kids being hit by cars, but adults often impulsively fall into harm's way when they are even slightly impaired and distracted with friends.

These stories are just a few I know about first hand; terrible events that happened to people

I know or that my kids know personally. I didn't look far and wide to find the most dramatic, outlandish stories. These are people who have touched our lives in one way or another and now have police records, are handicapped or dead because of one small fluky incident that went bad.

My point is that tragic stories stemming from drug and alcohol abuse are endless. Everyone you know has a story. If you avoid excessive partying and never walk alone at night, your odds of having a safe college experience are good! Remember, you're much safer with others and with a sharper brain!

This takes me back to the expression, "YOLO!" You do Only Live Once: let's not cut it short.

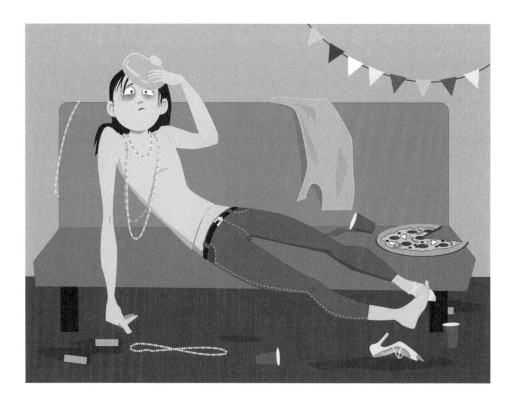

Am I drinking too much alcohol?

Unfortunately, some people rationalize excessive drinking in college as "a rite of passage" or believe it is something young people need to do to "get it out of their system." The reality is that you will be exposed to drinking in college. Alcohol use is widely accepted because it is legal at a certain age. But drinking can be extremely problematic at any age, legal or not.

The reality is that the excessive use of alcohol leads to strained relationships, lost or damaged valuables, violence, physical injury, car accidents, legal issues, promiscuity, unprotected sex, disease, pregnancy, rape, acute health issues and death.

What is binge drinking?

- For men, consuming five or more standard alcohol drinks within two hours.
- For women, consuming four or more standard alcoholic drinks within two hours.

What is a standard drink?

- 12 ounces of regular beer
- 8 to 9 ounces of malt liquor
- 5 ounces of wine
- 1 "shot" of 80-proof hard liquor

Research finds college students who binge drink regularly show damage to blood vessels that is similar to that of high blood pressure and cholesterol. This damage is known to increase risk of heart disease later in life.[29]

Ask yourself the following questions:

- Do you find your tolerance is way above everyone else's?
- Are you frequently "blacking out"? After a previous evening of drinking you can't recall events that occurred.
- Are you frequently "browning out"? After a previous evening of drinking you can't remember something until someone else brings it up.
- Are you frequently passing out because you are so sleepy from alcohol? This is a sign of poisoning from excessive alcohol intake, which is life threatening.
- Are you using alcohol as an escape from stress on a daily basis?
- Is your drinking interfering with the ability to fulfill your obligations at work, home or school?
- Is your behavior when using alcohol causing negative interaction with friends and family?
- Do you wonder if you are drinking too much? If so, you probably are!

One young woman simplified things in her own words: *"If you wake up and have anxiety about what you did or said last night, you drank TOO MUCH!"*

If you have concerns about your drinking, remember that all college campuses have resources to deal with your concerns, and all information about you will be kept confidential.

If you witness someone unconscious, unable to wake up, vomiting or exhibiting irregular breathing, don't be afraid to dial 911 for help!

So, with that said, CHEERS—in moderation!

Drugs

The reality is that many deadly drugs are out there on college campuses and available to you and your friends. Not one of those drugs is good for you. All of them are addictive and have the potential to cause great bodily harm or death. Please realize that just because a trusted friend has tried a drug and is doing all right, it could be a very different story for you.

Think about your mother, father, sister and brother, and imagine how devastated they would be if something happened to you. Drug abuse is serious. The Internet is full of stories about drug addiction and its tragic consequences. If this subject is something you are curious about, read, research and learn. I have touched on only a few types of drugs. I'm not an expert, but it doesn't take an expert to know that drugs harm and kill. Don't be a statistic, and don't allow yourself to rely on a drug for happiness.

A dear friend is dead in the blink of an eye. Is marijuana to blame?

A college freshman, whose teachers described him as "a really good kid with a bright future" was speeding, ran a stop sign, and hit a car containing a beautiful young mom and her 14-year-old twin daughters. The impact was so enormous that both the mom and one of the girls were thrown through the glass and out of their car. The young mom was killed instantly. One of the twins, a teen athlete, sustained severe injuries requiring surgeries and months of intensive medical treatment—all while she was mourning the death of her mom.

The widowed father of the family suffered the loss of the love of his life while struggling to hold the rest of the family together financially and emotionally. The three children in this family were without a mother at a point in their lives when they needed her the most. And the life of the young man who caused the accident was forever changed.

This 18-year-old driver had marijuana in his system. Did he smoke that day or 30 days earlier? Was he high or not? We may never know. We do know he faced vehicular homicide charges and will have to live with the guilt of his mistake for the rest of his life.

The mom of this story was a dear friend of mine. She will never be able to experience any of the joys that come with seeing her beloved children mature and grow to adulthood.

Drugs are illegal in most states, no matter what your age, and they do impair your judgment and actions. Be responsible and don't risk having a drug violation or, worse yet, a fatal accident. Lives are precious, and criminal charges will change the path of your life in a heartbeat. Instantly, the many roads that were once open for you will be defaced with detour signs everywhere, and the few routes available to you will often turn into dead ends.

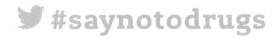 #saynotodrugs

Stimulant use and abuse

When you have procrastinated writing the 15-page paper that's due tomorrow, do you think about using prescription stimulants such as Adderal, Ritalin or Concerta so that you can stay up all night? Or maybe you tied one on last night and feel the need to take something that will keep you awake and alert for school today. What about popping a pill so that you can ace those finals? Do you have friends who swear they focus and play better in their sports when they are on Adderal? Have you heard that taking stimulant drugs is a great weight-loss technique? Or do you know people who simply use stimulants in large doses or drug mixtures to get high?

These are all reasons that kids seek out these drugs. They view the use of nonmedical stimulants as "no big deal." Young adults—and sometimes even their parents—often think that taking a Ritalin once in a while to gain a competitive edge is something that can be swept under the rug. Besides, why would anyone fear taking these pills when doctors widely prescribe them for so many young kids?

Unfortunately, nonmedical use of prescription stimulants is often a piece of a much larger problem. Research shows that those who seek out stimulants without a prescription often abuse alcohol and other elicit drugs. In addition, these powerful amphetamines are distributed with warnings that state they may cause "sudden death and serious cardiovascular adverse events" and have "a high potential for abuse."[30]

Stimulant prescription use has been very beneficial for many individuals who have had proper testing and diagnosis of conditions like ADHD. Unfortunately, the abuse of these stimulants by those that don't have a prescription may make it more difficult for physicians to prescribe stimulants in the future to those who really need them.

I have mixed emotions about this subject because I know great young adults who would not have made it through grade school without the medications that physicians prescribed for them. On the other hand, I hear from kids about how widely abused these drugs are in high schools and colleges. Many efforts are being made to educate doctors, school faculty members and parents about the risks and rewards of these drugs.

However, I have personally talked to mothers who have turned their cheek on instances where they know their kids get stimulants illegally. It has become a dangerous norm! It's important that you know parents would never support your amphetamine use if they knew the consequences of taking these drugs without a prescription.

The best guideline is: if a physician hasn't prescribed these medications for you, stay away from them! There are many reasons why they are not sold over the counter. Each patient is prescribed a dose that is safe for his or her particular situation and body weight. One pill could be 5 milligrams and another could be 50! It is not one size fits all in the world of prescription drugs!

What if you get caught with these controlled substances? If you feel you have a problem with attention or have difficulty focusing, see a physician and get a proper diagnosis. Other conditions besides ADHD can cause concentration issues.

If you do have prescriptions for stimulants, hide the pills and don't hand them out or sell them to others! If you possess them without a prescription or distribute these drugs to anyone, you may be charged with a felony. This would be a life changer!

"Molly": she sounds sweet, but she's deadly.

Most of you are familiar with the drug called "Ecstasy" or "Molly." We are talking about the drug MDMA or methylenedioxy-methylamphetamine. It's a synthetic, psychoactive drug that creates feelings of euphoria, higher energy, empathy toward others, and distortions in sensory and time perception.

Symptoms of an overdose of MDMA are high heart rate, high respiratory rate, and high blood pressure. These symptoms are hard to detect in nightclubs or concert halls, where the drug is often used. The drug causes a surge of serotonin, creating heightened mood. However, the aftereffects may include very negative feelings of confusion, depression, sleep problems, drug craving and anxiety.

The use of MDMA can result in failure of the liver, kidney or cardiovascular systems and even death. Moreover, the drug is often distributed after it has been combined with other unknown drugs or substances that may themselves be very harmful. Even worse results occur when these combinations are mixed with alcohol or marijuana. Bottom line: MDMA is deadly.[31]

The number of emergency room visits resulting from the use of MDMA has skyrocketed, and the death rate is continuing to rise. Any death from an overdose is a tragedy, but a young person dying from a one-time drug experiment is an unthinkable horror.

From prescription drugs to the use of heroin

A young man recently delivered this impactful message on national television:

> I lost six friends to overdoses in the last year. Out of 15 friends back at home, probably five of them are dead. It can happen to anybody and by doing it one time: one time can be too many![32]

I intended to end this chapter on drugs and alcohol with the preceding paragraph, and then I saw a special on TV about the epidemic of heroin use. I really didn't want to face this topic because it is so horrifying, and I didn't want to ignite any young person with a curiosity surrounding this poison! However, when one victim reiterated that if she had known any of the dangers of heroin, she never would have tried it, I realized knowledge is power.

In my naïve eyes, heroin was a drug that kids from really rough neighborhoods were exposed to. Only kids who had no love or guidance from their parents could possibly be involved with that kind of drug. This is not the case today.

Most commonly, people start with some kind of injury or surgery for which their family physician prescribes painkillers—opioids such as Vicoden, OxyContin and Percocet. Patients like the feeling of euphoria these meds give them, continue to crave them, and begin abusing them. Soon they can't get a hold of or afford the $80 pills anymore. They find out they can get heroin, a drug that affects the brain in the same way, readily and cheaply. From then on, life as they knew it, is no longer. The addiction to some of these drugs is beyond most people's comprehension. The devastation that can occur from trying some of these drugs just once can change you for a lifetime.

On national TV, a polished young man named Zach recently described his never-ending, heartbreaking battle with heroin. Zach had played hockey, football and lacrosse in high school and received a hefty scholarship to a prestigious prep school, followed by another scholarship to play lacrosse at a highly regarded college in the East. During his freshman year, he contracted Methicillin-resistant Staphlococcus aureus (MRSA), a painful infection for which he was given morphine. This drug elated and comforted him: he described feeling as if he were wrapped in a warm blanket. He soon was abusing pain medications at a cost of a thousand dollars a day. He quickly discovered that heroin is in the same class of drugs as morphine and is cheap, pure, and readily available.

What happened next? I'll let Zack tell you the rest of his tragic story:

> *Fast forward seven years: I didn't finish college, and now I'm hustling heroin on the streets. I don't know how to stop. I've sold everything I've owned—every computer, every Play Station. Everything of any value my parents owned is gone. I've been hospitalized, lived in sober houses, halfway houses, and state run programs, yet I'm still in the grips of addiction today. I don't want to continue, but I don't know if I could live a sober life.*
>
> *I do wake up saying I don't want to get high, but at the same time it's all I can think about. It literally consumes my mind. My body is craving it, my head is running with different schemes and ideas of how I can get it. I have felt good at the beginning of all my treatments—for maybe two, three months I'm feeling good and think, "I can beat this thing, I have it beat." But you never have this disease beat. It's just waiting. Death or jail. I don't see any other way out right now.*[33]

According to experts, this young man has rewired the reward pathways of his brain. He's at a point where his body and his brain tell him this drug is what he needs, and the situation starts to spiral out of control. His mother, sitting by her son's side and holding his hand, looked very weary and exhausted. She can't trust her son in her own home. She exclaimed tearfully, "I don't worry about whether he's taken 20 dollars anymore. I don't worry if a TV is missing. I do worry that I am going to get a phone call telling me that my son is dead."

Is addiction hopeless? Not always. Here is the story of Andrea, a beautiful, intelligent young woman who fell into the grips of heroin:

> *It all happened quickly: I didn't know what I was getting myself into. It started with marijuana, and when I realized that wasn't going to kill me, I forgot about any of the drug education I had had or any warning signs. I was really available to try anything.*
>
> *The first time I used heroin, it was being passed around at a party. I didn't even know what it was. By making that one choice, I lost everything in my life*

that mattered to me. I was emotionally depressed. I was doing things I never imagined. I didn't see any way out of this life.[34]

Eventually Andrea ended up in prison for forgery, a crime she committed to support her habit. She went to rehab sixteen times, and the sixteenth time she set her mind to finding the path to a drug-free life. She worked hard to put her life back together, fixing all the damage. Three years later she says, "It's possible."

For some, recovery is possible; for many, recovery seems incomprehensible. None of us know how our unique bodies will react to these substances. Trying it once is like playing Russian roulette.

Nicotine

I had no intention about reiterating the warnings we have all heard about tobacco and how its use can lead to heart disease, lung disease and cancer. However, I still see a lot of college-age kids puffing away desperately outside in subzero weather or sneaking chew whenever they have the opportunity. I have noticed that many guys can't just hang out without a wad of chew inside their lip, bulging like a chipmunk, storing his seeds! It's really the norm for these students to be spitting the smelly, muddy looking saliva into a water bottle while they are socializing or playing video games. Do you really find that attractive, ladies? You wouldn't find me kissing no spitting chipmunk!

Oral cancer is another health risk taken on from tobacco use and can be very serious, especially if it is not detected early on. According to the American Academy of Periodontology, tobacco use is a significant risk factor in developing periodontal disease, as well.[35]

Unhealthy gums can lead to many problems ranging from bad breath to losing your teeth! Nicotine use also slows the healing process after injury or surgery due to adverse effects on bone cells and blood vessels. Consequently, if you have some teeth extracted or any other type of surgery, you might take longer to heal than your nonsmoking friends.

Did you know that you might not be enjoying your food as much as you could be? Many individuals have reported their food tastes much better after they quit smoking. This change in sensation occurs because tobacco use often causes a dulled sense of taste and smell that is hard to realize until after you quit.

Finally, tobacco often stains those pearly whites. You

may not realize it, but your smile is a big part of your first impression. Take care of those teeth; you might get a second date! And if none of this makes an impression, tell the boys there are studies showing that cigarettes could significantly reduce penile erection. Yikes!

In all seriousness, tobacco is a stimulant and often helps some people feel more alert and focused. Students are constantly trying to find ways to boost their attention span. Unfortunately, there are too many unhealthy, tempting ways to do that. It's difficult to look ahead thirty years. Your able bodies can take a lot of abuse in the short term, but dangerous habits will often catch up with you and create devastating illness along with deep facial wrinkles later in life.

There is no question that nicotine is incredibly addictive and kicking the habit is extremely challenging. Once you have decided you are going to make this commitment to your health, make sure you have a good support system and a proven plan for success. You are worth it!

Contact your insurance to see if they provide smoking and tobacco cessation programs. Also you might go to: www.cancer.org/healthy/stayawayfromtobacco/guidetoquittingsmoking

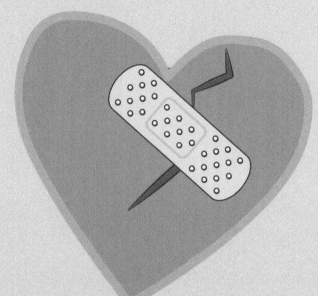

CHAPTER 9

Sex and
Relationships

"Don't be silly, wrap that willy!"

You have been hearing the words "protected sex" for years. The threats of pregnancy and sexually transmitted diseases have been described in your health classes since you were in grade school. The media has exploded with messages on these topics. However, have you really thought about how these issues affect *you*?

As I have mentioned before, my hope for you, my children, and my friends' and clients' children is that any young person's first experience with sex is filled with love, respect and commitment.

I have heard countless stories of teens and young adults who have lost their virginity in a few drunken moments or as a result of peer pressure. The entertainment industry floods our screens with primal, impulsive, passionate sex filled with "off the charts" ecstasy. Sex is portrayed as just another adventure with someone we have just met and really don't care if we ever see again. Really? Is that how all of us should look at sex—as if it were a casual hobby?

Serious emotional repercussions can result from having a sexual relationship before we are ready. You may not yet have even come close to having a sexual experience or, perhaps, you have had sex in your early teens. However, even if you are a sexually experienced young person, read on because I have important information for you, too!

Whatever your situation, if you are thinking about beginning a sexual relationship, keep thinking, and let your heart and brain guide you to a place and a decision with which you can live and feel comfortable. Guilt, shame and remorse can be devastating, and the aftermath of these emotions can stay with you indefinitely, often leading to depression.

The truth is that women have a hard time engaging in sexual activity without developing feelings or some sort of emotional connection with their partners. Post "hook-up" trauma is common among women who engage in casual sex and then realize the guy's not really interested in much else but the booty call. I am not saying the guys can't feel post "hook-up" trauma, too. Regardless of the situation, taking your clothes off with someone you don't know well often happens when you're under the influence—that brief time period when everything seems like a good idea and modesty seems to completely escape your mind!

Guilt for losing self-respect, guilt for using someone, guilt for breaching personal and religious moral beliefs, and fear of pregnancy and disease are enough to send anyone into a frenzy of negative emotion or depression. On the other hand, if you are with someone in a committed relationship and are able to talk and plan your activities and your lives, much less emotional and physical risk will be involved.

However, please remember that even if you are in a committed relationship, it is never all right for someone to pressure you into behaviors you are not ready for. If you find you are giving in as a result of pressure from your partner, then sex in that instance is a bad idea.

Sexually transmitted infections and disease

People are raised with many different beliefs and examples of how sex should fit into their lives. However, we all have one thing in common: every one of us is susceptible to the risks of unprotected sex. Perhaps you are someone who would not dare have unprotected sex. Or, perhaps, you are a risk taker and feel that the friends in your social group are immune to sexually transmitted diseases.

Whatever your attitudes or beliefs, I want you to close your eyes and pretend that you are nineteen years old, with your whole life in front of you, and a doctor has just told you that you have herpes, a disease that never goes away. What happens when you next meet someone you are serious about? What are the odds that this new love interest will give you a chance when you confide that you are infected with the incurable herpes virus? This bit of news is nothing other than devastating! On the other hand, if you do not have herpes, how can you be sure your partner is also disease free? You may say to yourself, "But he loves me! I know he hasn't been seeing anyone else, and he would never have sexual relations with me if he knew that he was carrying this virus!"

You have probably heard this before, but I'm going to tell you again: you are sleeping with anybody and everybody your partner has ever slept with! Use a condom and protect yourself from all of those people! Some individuals are infected with sexually transmitted diseases that are lifelong, yet they have no symptoms. Have you really heard about all the sexually transmitted infections and diseases out there and how devastating any one of them can be to your health and your intimate relationships? Let me list some of them: then, I hope, you will never ditch the condom again![36]

- Chancroid
- Chlamydia
- Cytomegalovirus (CMV)
- Genital warts
- Gonorrhea
- Hepatitis B
- Herpes
- HIV/Aids
- Human Papillomavirus (HPV)
- Intestinal parasites
- Molluscum Contagiosum
- Pelvic Inflammatory Disease
- Pubic lice (crabs)
- Scabies
- Syphilis
- Trichomoniasis (Trich)

Please remember that these diseases and infections are transmitted through oral sex and anal sex as well as through sexual intercourse.

It's important for me to note that many individuals who have been diagnosed with these sexually transmitted, incurable diseases have gone on to have fulfilling relationships, but not without complication. If you can, prevent the preventable!

For symptoms and more information visit:
http://www.plannedparenthood.org/health-topics/stds-hiv-safer-sex-101.htm

Pregnancy

If you are a young woman, close your eyes and pretend a doctor has just told you that you are pregnant. What is going through your mind? Are you considering an abortion? Are you considering adoption and wondering if you will have the strength to hand over your newborn to another family? Or do you picture yourself losing your independence and being responsible for another human being for the next twenty years—possibly with no involvement of the father?

If you choose abortion, will you always wonder what your child would have looked like or what kind of relationship the two of you would have had? Will the guilt of terminating a life haunt you for the rest of your life?

Do you know a guy who is being stupid and slutty? Tell him to close his eyes and pretend that a young woman has just told him that he is going to be a father. Ask him if he'll stand by her and spend the rest of his life with this woman and child? Or will he choose to leave her and be held responsible for making monthly payments in support of this child for the next eighteen years? Will either of you need to give up your dreams of going to graduate school or traveling the world? If you forget a condom or simply bank on the fact the birth control pills are working properly, you may be forced to make these kinds of life-changing decisions. All forms of birth control are capable of failing.

Once a pregnancy is a reality, there is no easy solution and, you can be assured, there will be some serious and demanding hardships along the way.

Take control over what you have control over. If you decide to have sex, your best bet is to use two forms of birth control!

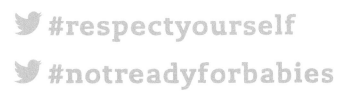

🐦 #respectyourself

🐦 #notreadyforbabies

Relationship tips from a college senior:

Relationships// 101

Tip 1. Don't be "THAT" drunk girl—yelling obnoxiously, dancing provocatively and stumbling over your own feet may seem fun at the time. Yes, we all want to have a great time—but waking up the next morning and not knowing what you said or did is the worst and can completely turn guys off. → You will regret it!

Tip 2. When you find someone you're interested in, whether you met them in the dorms or you sit next to them in your chemistry lab, introduce yourself. Be friendly. We are all in the same boat—people want to meet people! What's there to lose? → Go for it!

Tip 3. When you do find that special person, don't spend every night together. Living in a dorm and having a roommate gets exhausting. Would you want your roommate having someone sleep over every night? No. → Moderation.

Tip 4. You think you found your best friend, the love of your life, your soul mate. Great! Maybe you did. Don't block your friends out of your life. They will be there through thick and thin, and in all honesty, you don't know what will happen with your relationship. You're still young. → Keep the balance.

Tip 5. Keep each other on track. Study together. Work out together. Eat healthy together. Keeping one another motivated helps you both stay on top of your schoolwork and staying active/healthy → Be that dynamic duo!

Tip 6. You're both broke—it's reality. Go grocery shopping together and eat at home. You will save a lot of money and remember it's healthier than eating out! → Be smart with that pocket change of yours.

Tip 7. If he wants to have sex on the first date, don't! Trust me, he will have a lot more respect for you if you wait. It shows him you respect yourself and you don't just give your body out easily. → When you are ready—don't be silly, wrap that willy!

Breakups

Going through a breakup can be devastating and cause extreme mental anguish. Usually the timing of a breakup is the worst ever! The last thing you want to do is crawl in bed, miss your classes, fall behind in school, and increase your stress even more. Eating a carton of ice cream won't exactly put you in a good place either.

Tips for breakup survival[37]

- Have a good cry and express your feelings to a trusted friend.
- Don't get stuck in the blame game, dissecting the relationship and analyzing what went wrong. It's OK to soul search and be aware of unwanted behaviors, but now is the time to focus on how you are going to move forward.
- Cut off all contact with him. Communicating and trying to cross paths with him will just prolong the grieving process and cause unnecessary drama.
- Make some changes. Box up any reminders like pictures and gifts. Alter any routines or destinations that cause painful reminders of the relationship.
- Exercise and eat well even though you don't feel like it!
- Foster your independence. Have fun, but not **too** much fun! Stay single and enjoy your friends for a while. Prove to yourself that it's OK to *not* be in a relationship.
- If you see him at a party and have had a little bit too much to drink, don't go home with him. Avoid the temptation at all cost!
- Don't dwell on his latest hook-up. Chances are it meant nothing and it's his only way to cope and make himself feel better temporarily! His way of grieving could be very different from yours!
- Know in your heart that if you are meant to be together, it will most likely only happen if you completely let him go. Experience other relationships and come back after more personal growth and maturity.

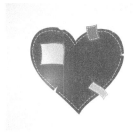

Here is a great love story, which demonstrates the growth and maturity that comes from college relationships—the breakups and heartaches.

I was 14 and I fell hard for the cute, fun boy in my math class. We had become incredibly serious at such a young age. We were inseparable. Cody was my best friend and the love of my life, so I thought. We actually talked about marriage and our future together. He was 100 percent committed to me and treated me like a princess.

But my feelings took a turn soon after I met Kyle—the charismatic, bad boy that grabbed every girl's attention. He flirted with me incessantly in chemistry class and soon won me over. Consequently, my future with Cody was over. I broke his heart into tiny little pieces. He burned every love letter and photo we shared. Our memories and our future were destroyed.

My relationship was exciting with Kyle. I had landed this gorgeous guy every other girl wanted, and he was fun with a capital F! But as time went on, the fairy tale turned disastrous. He played with my heart, was dishonest and didn't treat me the way I knew I should be treated. For some reason, I couldn't let go. After three years of this rollercoaster relationship, we were off to different colleges and found the courage to move on from each other.

Now I was a freshman in college and single. I hated being single! I dated around a little, but soon latched on to the first guy who was boyfriend material. We stayed together about a year, but I ended it because of his alcohol dependency and emotional abuse. I never realized how toxic alcohol could be to relationships.

My second serious college relationship lasted two years and was healthy and honest. We pushed each other to be our best. I really thought he might be "the one." However, his home was in Canada and our lives were headed in two different directions. After we split, I realized I was never completely myself around him. As painful as it was, I knew it was for the best.

A few months later, spring semester of my senior year ended and I moved home with a broken heart. My neighbor was having people over and invited me for a beer. I walked in, and seated on the couch was Cody, my first love.

For the first time in seven years we were both single and had an opportunity to hang out together and catch up.

All the old feelings came flooding back. I understood why I compared everyone I ever dated to Cody. By the end of the evening, I knew I wanted him back. He was now a man, but the same honest, sincere person I fell in love with at 14 years old. Cody, however, hadn't forgotten the tremendous pain I had caused him. For that reason, we took things slowly. I had a lot of convincing to do!

The love Cody and I share now is something so much more than anything I had ever experienced. Cody has shown me a love everyone deserves, a love so real.

Looking back on the ups and downs, the laughter and tears, the joy and heartbreak, I now know that college was an important time for my emotional growth. I needed to play the field, kiss a few frogs, and experience some heartache to realize the qualities I wanted and needed in a life partner.

Today we are planning our life together, and there is no hesitation, question or regret about where I have been and where I am headed in the future. I do believe everything happens for a reason. When times are tough, it sometimes takes months or even years to find the silver lining. But in the end clarity usually emerges.

—Shelby, age 22

CHAPTER 10
Sexual Assault

It's never, ever OK.

It's just in the movies that a scary masked man hides in your home waiting to attack, right? Here is another personal story that a beautiful, young woman—a courageous survivor—told me recently:

Never in a million years would you think this would happen to you, EVER!

In the middle of an afternoon in January of my sophomore year, I walked into my apartment, flipped on the TV, and made myself a bowl of soup. After I ate, I sat down and started working on my homework. When I looked up, I saw a man wearing a ski mask and standing in front of me with a knife in his hand. I tried to scream, but nothing came out of my mouth. Nothing. He waved the knife in my face, then grabbed me and dragged me into the back bedroom. He tied my hands with a gymnastics hair ribbon that was sitting on my dresser and put tape across my eyes.

He then started rummaging through the apartment and kept asking, "Where's the money? Where's the money?" I kept saying, "We're college kids. We don't have any!" He found nothing of significant value anywhere—no money, no jewelry—and he kept getting madder. He was very angry and very drunk. I could smell the alcohol on his breath.

I started to hyperventilate. I couldn't breathe and thought, "I'm going to pass out." I started to pray, asking God for help and strength and saying "I don't want to die. I'm too young, and what's my mother going to do?" Within a second, I felt calm and at peace from the top of my head to the tips of my toes. I started breathing normally. I said to myself, "If he stabs me, it is not going to hurt, and I'm not going to bleed, either." I knew I was going to wake up the next day.

Then he raped me. I couldn't fight back because my hands were tied and I still had tape on my face. He started to leave and told me to stay put. He said he would be back in a few minutes and if I tried to get help or call anyone, he would know. He did come back and went in and out, taking things from the apartment.

When he left the last time, I tried to get the tape off my eyes by rubbing it on the corner of the dresser. I waited for what seemed like an eternity to make sure he was gone for good—maybe 30 minutes to an hour. Then I got the tape off my face and broke the tape and ribbon that was on my wrists. In doing so, I actually damaged a nerve in my hand.

I was calm until I got to my neighbor's. However, once I saw another person, I started screaming. My neighbor called the police. They took me to a hospital to do testing for DNA. I also had to take a morning-after pill to prevent pregnancy.

My mom and dad were in California, so my sister drove back to Minnesota to stay with me. I soon flew to California for a couple of weeks to be with my parents. When I got back, the stories were insane. I walked into the student center with my boyfriend, and you could have heard a pin drop. It was a small college, and everyone knew what had happened. All eyes stared at me. I looked down, and Bob said, "Don't do that. Hold your head up. You didn't do anything wrong." I realized that what had happened was either going to ruin me or I could rise from this.

I can honestly say that this experience has made me who I am, and I am a better person because of it. It's important to surround yourself with people who will support and help you. I wasn't going to let this beat me. There is nothing you can go through that is so horrible that you can't recover from it and become better.

Sometimes young adults get to the point where they tell themselves, "I just can't do it anymore." But you can. You just have to find the people who love and support you.

I got a great counselor who helped me realize this experience hadn't been my fault. I hadn't done anything to cause it to happen. I just was an unfortunate victim of a really bad circumstance. When something like that happens to you, you are at a fork in a road, and you can let it control you or you can control it. I wasn't going to let this one bad day define who I was.

—Dani, age 19

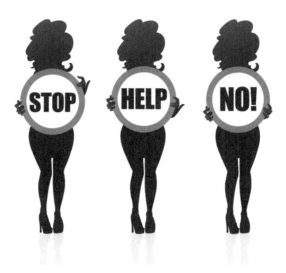

Date rape

Most moms feel their kids are safe when surrounded by good friends. In many cases that's true. However, a mom I know told me the following story, which illustrates how quickly bad things can happen even in familiar places and why friends should stick together.

> Not long ago, I was having a conversation with my daughter Kelly, who is a college student. The subject of date rape came up. She looked at me with horror and said, "Mom, I know beyond a shadow of a doubt that I was given the date rape drug about six months ago!"
>
> I said, "What? And you never told me this?" I was shocked. I thought my child told me everything.
>
> Kelly said, "I didn't want to tell you because I knew you would constantly worry about me. Remember last summer when you found me sleeping on the porch early one morning—and I told you the front door had been locked when I came home the previous evening and I hadn't wanted to awaken you to get into the house? That was the night."
>
> At that moment, I froze and was praying she hadn't been raped or hurt.

"I was with a friend at a bar near the college campus," Kelly said. "Two guys bought us a couple of shots, and that's the last thing I remember. I found out later I had passed out with my head on a table. Two girls came and somehow got me out of there and found somebody in my phone contacts to pick me up and get me from campus to my home safely. I was dropped off in my driveway and stumbled onto the porch where I passed out."

"The next day, I couldn't believe what had happened to me. There is no way I would have had a reaction like that after two drinks. It was so scary, Mom! I am so thankful those girls helped me. Who knows where I might have ended up otherwise?"

College administrators want their campuses to be safe and do try to promote awareness and implement safety measures. However, sexual assault and date rape are very prevalent on college campuses. When you hear the term rape, you generally think of a man hiding in the bushes ready to attack on the walking trail or someone breaking into your house. However, **about 85 to 90 percent of sexual assaults reported by college women are perpetrated by someone known to the victim, and about half occur on a date.**[38]

Most women don't label an incident as rape if a weapon is not used, alcohol is involved, and no signs of physical abuse are present. For this reason, many rapes are not reported. As few as 5 percent of attempted and completed rapes of college students are reported to campus administrators or law enforcement officers, according to a study completed by the U.S. Department of Justice.[39]

The National Institute of Justice defines a sexual assault as a wide range of unwanted behaviors—up to but not including penetration—that are attempted or completed against a victim's will or when a victim cannot consent because of age, disability or the influence of alcohol or drugs. Sexual assault may involve actual or threatened physical force, use of weapons, coercion, intimidation or pressure, and may include:[40]

- Intentional touching of the victim's genitals, anus, groin or breasts
- Voyeurism (spying on people when they are undressing or engaging in sexual intimacy.)
- Exposure to exhibitionism
- Undesired exposure to pornography
- Public display of images taken in a private context when the victim was unaware

Rape

Most states currently define rape as a nonconsensual oral, anal or vaginal penetration of the victim by body parts or objects using force, threats of bodily harm or by taking advantage of a victim who is incapacitated or otherwise incapable of giving consent. Incapacitated may include mental or cognitive disability, self-induced or forced intoxication, status as minor, or any other condition defined by law that voids an individual's ability to give consent.[41]

The first two years of college and the first months of school seem to show higher incidents of sexual assault.[42] Many students act like caged animals when they hit the campus in the fall of their freshman year. The anticipation of independence and freedom is the best feeling in the world, and the fun begins. Alcohol use has been identified as the highest risk factor for sexual assault. Young women who drink too much put themselves in harm's way. In addition, their intoxication coupled with a young man's intoxication can be trouble with a capital T.

This leads us to the topic of sororities and fraternities. Being a member of the campus Greek system has wonderful benefits. You instantly have a large group of friends, you are required to keep up your grades, and the social gatherings and functions are endless.

My best friends today are young women I met in my sorority. Despite the large campus of the college I attended, the sorority gave me an instant feeling of belonging and kinship. There was always someone to answer questions or encourage me when school was tough, and the academic motivation was greatly enhanced. However, studies show that incidents of sexual assault are higher among those who have a sorority membership.[43]

Would I recommend joining a sorority? Absolutely! However, if alcohol or drugs are being used at any parties on campus or off campus, be careful. Impairment increases the risk of sexual assault.

Also, studies show that those who have numerous sexual partners after entering college are more at risk.[44] Why? Perhaps the more young women open themselves up to sex, the more young men might expect them to put out. This is never ever an acceptable excuse for guys to push the limits, but the truth is, it happens. It's wrong, and the consequences can be devastating for a very long time.

Whatever your choices are regarding sexual intimacy, it is safest and most respectful to yourself to share those moments with someone who respects and cares about you in a committed, loving, trusting relationship. That's my strong opinion!

Let me spell out in bold letters there is no implication here that "at risk" young women are **EVER** in any way responsible for a sexual crime, but identifying risk factors is one way we can help prevent assaults.

Tips for self-defense[45]

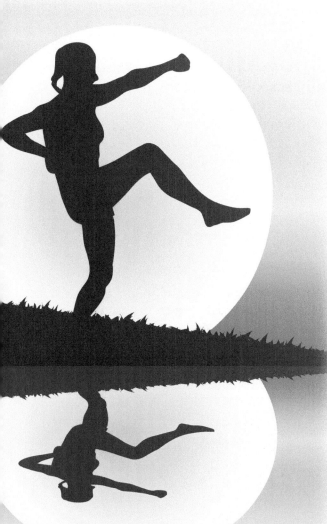

- Educate yourself and have a plan. Watch some self-defense videos on YouTube or take a self-defense workshop. Take the time to envision your plan of action for different scenarios. Prepare and empower the mind and body to take action with strength and courage instead of weakness.

- Focus on your surroundings and not your gadgets. Act confident and assured. Don't give predators opportunities to catch you off guard when you're digging through your purse or distracted by your phone. If you sense someone is following you, move into a safer area like a store or business. If this isn't possible, look him in the eye or even ask him a question to give him the message you are unafraid and will stick up for yourself if you need to. Rapists are weaker than you think. They don't like to deal with strong, confident women, especially those that have looked him in the face and can identify him in a line-up!

- Don't forget to keep your home safe. Lock your doors and keep the garage shut day and night. If you are on ground level, sleeping with the windows open can be dangerous, especially on a college campus!

- Be car smart. Women can be especially vulnerable in parking ramps, parking lots and secluded hallways, even in their own apartment buildings! Don't unlock your car with the remote until you are close to it. You don't want a bad guy to beat you to it! Hold your keys between your knuckles in case you need a weapon. As soon as you get in your car, lock the door and move on. Sitting in a parked car, distracted by your phone could make you a target.

  If you see a van parked next to your car, be aware of the possibility of a predator transporting you into it and get in on the passenger side instead. Remember safety in numbers. Stay alert, move quickly or better yet, take a shuttle when possible after dark or have someone walk with you to your car or building entrance if you can.

- Be careful on spring break! When you are traveling, you are more vulnerable. It's easy to get caught off guard in new and distracting surroundings. Lock your hotel room, and don't answer the door if you're not absolutely sure who it is! Be careful roaming the halls alone, especially at night. Don't set your drinks down at the nightclub, and be leery of any guys you meet that you don't know! Girlfriends go together, stay together, and leave together. This rule cannot be broken!

- Fighting is OK and sometimes the only way out! Statistics show those who fight off an attack verbally and physically are far more likely to get away. Rapists hate a fight! That is where your plan of action will benefit you. There must be no hesitation or pleading with this monster who will never be swayed by rational talk and decision-making the way you are use to. Hurt him badly and run! Acting with violence goes against everything you have been taught, but you not only have to fight, you have to fight dirty! Poke him in the eyes, karate chop him in the side of the neck, kick him in the knees or groin and hope he buckles. Hurting him badly enough to slow him down may give you your chance to get away.

- Don't let him take you away. You do not want to get in his vehicle! Your chances of injury and death increase dramatically if he is allowed to bring you to a new location. His threatening you with a gun should not even prevent you from putting up a fight. Rarely will a perpetrator actually use the weapon. They would rather not alert others to the scene! And even if he does, his chances of killing you are unlikely.

- Don't succumb to date rape even though the lines can be fuzzy, with or without alcohol! Anyone who tries to pressure you into doing things you are not ready for is not a person you want to continue hanging out with. There should be no worry about disappointing your date or pissing him off! The words "no" and "stop" are nonnegotiable! If he ignores your words, tell him not to "rape" you, in hopes he recognizes what he is doing and backs off. If that doesn't work, fight as though he is a stranger in a dark ally.

- Be aware of men who go out of their way to talk to you. It's rare that a man without ulterior motives would ask a woman who is alone for help or for favors. If someone comes to your car door or tries to talk to you about anything in a parking lot, don't let your guard down. The fear of being rude can increase your vulnerability and get you into a lot of trouble. Caution is the key! Rudeness is not a problem!

- Go with your gut. Follow your instincts in any unexpected situation. You can have all the education in the world, but your intuition is powerful.

If you are ever a victim of sexual assault and are hesitant to tell officials, remember there are options for reporting incidents confidentially and anonymously while deciding whether to file an official report. The Rape, Abuse and Incest National Network (Rainn) offers an anonymous online hotline available to victims of sexual assault: www.rainn.org or 1-800-656-hope.

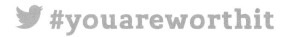 #youareworthit

Conclusion

Many of the days you spend in college will, most likely, be among the best days of your life. During these years, you will be able to explore endless opportunities. Your newly developed strength as an individual will allow you to make positive, independent decisions. Your social experiences will help you define who you are and what types of people you wish to make a part of your future. You will probably make many friends—some, perhaps, for a lifetime. Your newfound wisdom, growth and maturity will allow you to develop adult relationships with your parents, their friends, and their colleagues: those who once may have been policing you may now want to befriend you or hire you!

If you stay aware, listen to the voice of reason in your head, surround yourself with people who have positive behaviors, get support when you need it, make time for fun, stay on top of your responsibilities, and take care of your body, you WILL have an outstanding college experience. This unique time of learning is the beginning of the rest of your life, so savor every moment. A positive path creates a positive future.

Not sure you know what you want to do with your life? Most people don't, but your true purpose could be sitting right in front of you and you may not even realize it. Identify your interests by asking yourself what books and websites you have looked at, what hobbies have you been drawn to, and what topics you like talking about. Create a visual aid of your interests by making a collage or writing a list. As you look at the visual, key in on your top interests and imagine yourself in those fields with that lifestyle. How does it fit your personality and values? Would sitting at a desk for hours at a time drive you crazy? Does interacting with people all day pump you up? Would working into the evenings or traveling often be a conflict if you value family time?

You have plenty of time to figure it all out. And like many things in life, it can be trial and error. Finding your passion and your purpose leads to happiness and contentment and being at peace with your decisions is good for your mind and body. Believe in yourself, and don't ever give up!

If you can imagine it, you can achieve it; if you can dream it, you can become it.

—William Arthur Ward

NOTES

1.   Dalton Conley, "Wired for Distraction: Kids and Social Media," Time, 21 Feb. 2011, http://www.content. time.com/time/magazine/article/0,9171,2048363,00.html (accessed 22 Jan. 2014).

2.   Annie Murphy Paul, "You'll Never Learn!" Slate, 3 May 2013, http://www.slate.com/articles/health_and_ science/science/2013/05/multitasking_while_studying_divided_attention_and_technological_gadgets.html (accessed 5 Feb. 2014).

3.   Larry D. Rosen, "iDisorder," Dr. Larry Rosen: Books, 2012, http://www.drlarryrosen.com/topics/books/ (accessed 4 Apr. 2014).

4.   Larry D. Rosen, iDisorder (New York: Palgrave Macmillan, 2013), 207.

5.   Shirley Archer "Digital Distractions," Idea Fitness Journal (June 2013), 49.

6.   Academic Resource Center, "Effective Time Management," Duke University, http//www.duke.edu/arc/ documents/Effective%20time%20management.pdf (accessed 7 May 2013).

7.   The Center for Teaching and Learning, "Time Management," Stanford University, http//www.stanford.edu/ dept/CTL/Students/studyskills/time-manage.pdf (accessed 7 May 2013).

8.   University of Warwick, "Sleep Deprivation Doubles Risks of Obesity in Both Children and Adults," ScienceDaily, 13 July 2006, http://www.sciencedaily.com/releases/2006/07/060713081140.htm (accessed 21 May 2014).

9.   Noran Clinic Sleep Center, "Sleep Disorders," Noran Neurological Clinic, 2012, http://www.noranclinic. com/sleepcenter/sleep_disorders.html (accessed 21 May 2014).

10.   American Heart Association, "Sugars and Carbohydrates," American Heart Association: Getting Healthy, http://www.heart.org/HEARTORG/GettingHealthy/nutritionDietGoals/sugars-and-carbohydrates_ UCM_303296_article.jsp (accessed 20 Feb. 2014).

11.   U.S. Department of Agriculture and U.S. Department of Health and Human Services, "Dietary Guidelines for Americans 2010," Health.gov, http://www.health.gov/dietaryguidelines.dga/2010/DietaryGuidelines2010. pdf (accessed 20 Feb. 2014).

12.   Harvard Medical School, "High Calcium Intake from Supplements Linked to Heart Disease in Men," Harvard Health Publications: Harvard Health Blog, 6 Feb. 2013, http://www.health.harvard.edu/blog/high-calcium-intake-from-supplements-linked-to-heart-disease-in-men201302065861 (accessed 20 Feb. 2014).

13.   Ibid.

14.   Weill Cornell Medical College: Iris Cantor Women's Health Center, "Avoid the Energy Rollercoaster," Women's Nutrition Connection, no. 12G, 1, 5.

15.   Cedric X. Bryant and Daniel J. Green, Eds., ACE Lifestyle & Weight Management Coach Manuel: The Ultimate Resource for Fitness Professionals (San Diego: American Council on Exercise, 2011), 142-143.

16.   Melina Jampolis, "Expert Q & A, "CNN: Health, 9 Oct. 2009, http://www.cnn.com/2009/HEALTH/ expert.q.a/10/08/healthy.snacks.dorm.jamolis/index.html (accessed 2013).

17.   David L. Katz, Dr. David Katz's Flavorful Diet: Use Your Tastebuds to Lose Pounds and Inches with this Scientifically Proven Plan" (New York: Rodale Inc., 2007).

18. Biray Alsac-Seitz, "Smart Apps for Smart Appetites," IDEA Food and Nutrition Tips (Nov-Dec. 2012), 21.

19. Diana Rodriguez, "The Truth about Freshman 15," Everyday Health, 16 Dec. 2011, http://everydayhealth. com/college-health/avoid-the-freshman-15?xid=tw_everydayhealth_20111216_college (accessed 4 Dec. 2012).

20. U.S. Department of Health and Human Services, "Be Active Your Way Blog," Health.gov, 24 Oct. 2012, http://www.health.gov/paguidelines/how-much-daily-exercise-is-best-for-weight-loss.aspx (accessed 20 Feb. 2014).

21. American Heart Association "Physical Activity Improves Quality of Life," American Heart Association: Getting Healthy, 22 Mar. 2013, http://www.heart.org/HEARTORG/GettingHealthy/PhysicalActivity/ StartWalking/Physical-activity-improves-quality-of-life_UCM_307977_Article.jsp (accessed 1 Mar. 2014).

22. Mayo Clinic Staff. "Eating Disorders, Symptoms," Mayo Clinic: Diseases and Conditions, 8 Feb 2012, http://www.mayoclinic.org/diseases-conditions/eating-disorders/basics/symptoms/con-20033575 (accessed 21 Feb. 2014).

23. Ibid.

24. Mayo Clinic Staff, "Eating Disorders: Coping and Support," Mayo Clinic: Diseases and Conditions, 8 Feb. 2012, http://www.mayoclinic.com/health/eating-disorders/DS00294/DSECTION=coping%2Dand%2Dsupport (accessed 21 Feb. 2014).

25. American Psychiatric Association, Diagnostic and Statistical Manual of Mental Disorders, 4th ed. (Arlington, VA: American Psychiatric Publishing, 1994).

26. Ibid.

27. Ibid.

28. Jennifer Acosta Scott, "College Life: 10 Ways to Reduce Stress," Everyday Health, 17 Mar. 2012, http:// www.everydayhealth.com/college-health/college-life-10-ways-to-reduce-stress.aspx (accessed 4 Dec. 2012).

29. Paddock, Catharine, "Binge Drinking in College Years May Raise Risk for Heart Disease," Medical News Today, 24 Apr. 2013, http://www.medicalnewstoday.com/articles/259560.php (accessed 21 Feb. 2014).

30. Amelia M. Arria and Robert L. Dupont, "Nonmedical Prescription Stimulant Use Among College Students: Why We Need to Do Something and What We Need to Do," J. Addict Dis. 2010 October: 29(4): 417-426. Doi:1 0.1080/10550887.2010.509273, excerpted, National Institute of Health: NIH Public Access Author Manuscript, http://www.ncbi.nlm.nih.gov/pmc/articles/PMC2951617/ (accessed 21 Aug. 2013).

31. National Institute on Drug Abuse, "DrugFacts: MDMA (Ecstasy or Molly)," National Institute on Drug Abuse & Addiction, Sept. 2013, http://www.drugabuse.gov/publications/drugfacts/mdma-ecstasy-or-molly (accessed 14 Sept. 2013).

32. "Dirty Little Secret in the Suburbs," 10 June 2013, Katie, (KSTP).

33. Ibid.

34. Ibid.

35. American Academy of Periodontology, "Gum Disease Risk Factors," American Academy of Periodontology: PERIO.ORG, 2014, http://www.perio.org/consumer/risk-factors (accessed 21 Feb. 2014).

36. Planned Parenthood Federation of America Inc., "Sexually Transmitted Diseases (STD's)," Planned Parenthood Care No Matter What: Health Info and Services, 2014, http://www.plannedparenthood.org/health-topics/stds-hiv-safer-sex-101.htm (accessed 22 May 2014).

37. RooGirl staff, "9 Steps to Mending a Broken Heart," RooGirl: Sex and Love, 11 Apr. 2013, http://www.

roogirl.com/9-steps-to-mending-a-broken-heart/ (accessed 22 Feb 2014).

38. National Institute of Justice, "Most Victims Know Their Attacker," National Institute of Justice: Sexual Assault on Campus, 1 Oct. 2008, http://www.nij.gov/topics/crime/rape-sexual-violence/campus/pages/know-attacker.aspx (accessed 21 Feb. 2014).

39. Ibid.

40. Ibid.

41. Ibid.

42. National Institute of Justice, "Factors That Increase Sexual Assault," National Institute of Justice: Sexual Assault on Campus," 1 Oct. 2008, http://www.nij.gov/topics/crime/rape-sexual-violence/campus/pages/increased-risk.aspx (accessed 21 Feb. 2014).

43. Ibid.

44. Ibid.

45. Sheri Hosale, "14 Self-defense Tips Every Woman Should Know," Roogirl: Everyday life, 17 Apr. 2013, http://www.roogirl.com/14-self-defese-tips-every-woman-should-know/ (accessed 22 Feb. 2014).

ADDITIONAL REFERENCES

Connie Brichford (March 17, 2010). "Binge Drinking: Alcohol Abuse on Campus," *Everyday Health,* 17 Mar. 2010, http://www.everydayhealth.com/college-health/binge-drinking-alcohol-abuse-on-campus.aspx (accessed 5 Dec. 2012).

Evelyn Tribole and Elyse Resch, Intuitive Eating: A Revolutionary Program That Works (New York: Martins Press 2003).

Heather M. Kargane "Sexual Assault on Campus: What Colleges and Universities Are Doing About It," *U.S. Department of Justice Office of Justice Programs: National Institute of Justice,* 5 Dec. 2005, http://www.ojp.usdoj.gov/nij (24 Apr. 2013).

Maya Paul and Lawrence Robinson, "Healthy Fast Food: Tips for Making Healthier Fast Food Choices," *Helpguide.org,* http://www.helpguide.org/life/fast_food_nutrition.htm (accessed 23 May 2014).

Mayo Clinic Staff. "Dietary Fats: Know Which Types to Choose," *Mayo Clinic Healthy Lifestyle: Nutrition and Healthy Eating,* Feb. 2011, http://www.mayoclinic.org/fat/art-20045550 (accessed 10 Jan. 2014).

Mayo Clinc Staff, "Dietary Fiber: Essential for a Healthy Diet," *Mayo Clinic Healthy Lifestyle: Nutrition and Healthy Eating,* 17 Nov. 2012, http://www.mayoclinic.org/fiber/art-20043983 (accessd 15 Jan. 2014).

Mayo Clinic Staff, "Sodium: How to Tame Your Salt Habit," *Mayo Clinic Healthy Lifestyle: Nutrition and Healthy Eating,* 30 May 2013, http://www.mayoclinic.org/sodium/art-20045479?p=1 (accessed 7 Jan. 2014).

Mayo Clinic Staff, "Trans Fat Is Double Trouble for Your Heart Health," *Mayo Clinic Diseases and Conditions: High Cholesterol,* 6 May 2011, http://www.mayoclinic.org/diseases-condition/high-blood-cholesterol/in-depth/trans-fat/art-20046114 (accessed 10 Jan. 2014).

Michelle Annese, "17 Self-Defense Tips for College Dorm and Campus Safety," *College Tidbits,* 12 Mar. 2009, http://collegetidbits.com/wordpress/2009/03/12/17-self-defense-tips-for-dorm-and-campus-safety/ (accessed 22 Feb. 2014).

National Institute of Justice, "Certain Self-Defense Actions Can Decrease Risk," *Office of Justice Programs: National Institute of Justice,* 1 Oct. 2008, http://www.nij.gov/topics/crime/rape-sexual-violence/campus/pages/decrease-risk.aspx (accessed 21 Feb. 2014).

National Institute of Justice, "Rape and Sexual Violence," *Office of Justice Programs: National Institute of Justice,* 26 Oct. 2010, http://www.nij.gov/topics/crime/rape-sexual-violence/pages/welcome.aspx (accessed 21 Feb. 2014).

Serena Gordon,"Even in Young Adults, Binge Drinking May Harm Circulation," *Health Day,* 23 Apr. 2013, http://consumer.healthday.com/general-health-information-16/alcohol-abuse-news-12/even-in-young-adults-binge-drinking-may-harm-circulation-675676.html (accessed 23 May 2014).

Shereen Jegtvig, "Food Fight: Butter Vs. Margarine" *About.com: nutrition,* http://nutrition.about.com/od/milkdairyandcalcium/a/butter_or_marg.htm (accessed 23 May 2014).

CPSIA information can be obtained at www.ICGtesting.com
Printed in the USA
LVOW01s0705030615

440973LV00011B/47/P